Strategic Planning, Marketing, and Evaluation for Nursing Education and Service

Carolyn Feher Waltz

Susan Bond Chambers

Nan B. Hechenberger

Pub. No. 15–2282

National League for Nursing

Copyright © 1989
National League for Nursing
10 Columbus Circle, New York, NY 10019

ISBN 0-88737-444-1

The views expressed in this publication represent the views of the authors and do not necessarily reflect the official views of the National League for Nursing.

Printed in the United States of America

Contents

Contributors

Susan Bond Chambers, MBA, is Senior Evaluation Specialist, Office of Employment Development, City of Baltimore, Baltimore, MD

Nan B. Hechenberger, PhD, RN, is Professor and Dean, University of Maryland School of Nursing, Baltimore, MD.

Carolyn Feher Waltz, PhD, RN, FAAN, is Professor and Coordinator for Evaluation, University of Maryland School of Nursing, Baltimore, MD.

Preface

This book is meant to serve as a comprehensive resource for nurses involved in the design and implementation of strategic planning, marketing, and evaluation. It is a pragmatic account of the principles involved in such efforts and provides readers with a conceptual and operational basis for carrying out these processes. Our own experiences in nursing and other health fields guided the selection of topics and examples, resulting in the inclusion of content, strategies, and techniques with direct applicability for the implementation of the title processes in a variety of settings. This book has direct applicability for nursing administrators as well as nursing students in basic and advanced nursing administration courses. Graduate nurses with varying levels of preparation and experience will find the book a valuable resource for expanding their knowledge of administration as well as guiding their conduct in planning, marketing, and evaluation in education and service settings.

The authors assume that readers have little or no background in administration. Consequently, the book develops and details concepts and principles, with many step-by-step examples provided throughout the text. In addition, for the more sophisticated reader, strategies and techniques for operationalizing these concepts that are not found in other nursing books are provided here.

Reference citations are mainly comprehensive summaries of literature in a general area, rather than lists of individual books and articles.

Carolyn Feher Waltz
Susan Bond Chambers
Nan B. Hechenberger

1

Strategic Planning

Nan B. Hechenberger

Today, there is renewed significance for both the theory and practice of administration in complex organizations. The environment for the health care industry and for higher education mandates an entirely new character to the administration of nursing programs in practice and education. The administration of these programs needs to reflect conscious efforts in planning their development, relating process to outcome, and seeking an optimum return, both quantitatively and qualitatively, from limited resources.

RATIONALE FOR STRATEGIC PLANNING, MARKETING, AND EVALUATION

During the last half century, we have moved from a depression when few people could afford health care, particularly hospitalization, through a period when most working people were covered by some type of health insurance plan, and into an era of phenomenal growth in the health care industry that has been fueled, in large part, by the birth of the Medicare system. Currently, the industry is in a period of upheaval as a result of what is perhaps the most visible aspect so far of a pervasive reshaping of health care delivery—the Prospective Payment System (PPS).

For nurses, the implications of the PPS have been myriad. Hospitals, pressured to reduce operating budgets, have responded in some instances by the short-sighted cutting of nursing staff. In other instances, they have recognized that high-caliber professional nursing staff, in fact, can be cost effective by providing the quality of care that reduces complications, shortens hospital stays, and prevents readmissions. The major problem in health care today—cost—is nursing's greatest advantage. Studies demonstrate that nursing is one of the most basic cost containment tools available to the health care delivery system (Fagin, 1982; NLN, 1984).

The development of new technologies, the increasing number of the elderly and chronically ill, and the shifting focus toward alternative health care delivery systems emphasizing health promotion and hospital case mixes that consist of more critically ill patients requiring highly technical and continuous nursing care all step up the demand for nurses who can make well-informed, discriminating decisions and clinical judgments in stressful, complex-care situations. These are nurses who can function more autonomously to provide a full range of nursing services, including direct patient care, patient education, and counseling. Changes in corporate structure, contract services, and payment mechanisms include more nurses in administration, management, and consultation. In a health care economy impelled by the need to restrain costs, it is critical that nursing-service administrators be expert managers. Insufficient education in management often places these nurses at a serious disadvantage and compromises their ability to deliver quality nursing care. It is essential, therefore, to elevate the managerial expertise of these nurse administrators responsible for large budgets and complex management systems.

Nurses need to be able to compete with each other and with other health care professionals by using the factors associated with cost-effectiveness to advantage in gaining more professional responsibility and independence. The overriding concern of nursing, however, needs to be quality, because of the danger that resources will be withheld to contain cost. Nursing needs to emerge as the link between cost and quality in health care. The nurse is the institution's major marketing resource; he or she is seen by the public as the coordinator of care and patient advocate who guides the consumer through a complex and impersonal health care labyrinth.

In addition to being impacted by trends in the health care industry, administrators in schools of nursing, for the first time in 30 years, must respond to environmental conditions in a buyer's market, rather than a seller's market. The changing practice market, greater educational opportunities for women, and changing demographics in our society have led to declining enrollments in schools of nursing. In addition to declining enrollments, deteriorating facilities, smaller state appropriations, fewer federal dollars, and more competition for private dollars imply a different approach to the recruitment, retention, and graduation of nursing students, and to the overall administration and governance of schools of nursing. Unpopular as the notion may be in some quarters, it is time for a healthy dose of corporate discipline to be imposed upon the academy!

The need for strategic planning and data-based decision making is crucial if schools of nursing are to survive, compete, and progress in educating health care professionals, contribute to the generation and transmission of new nursing knowledge, and provide services to the community and to the profession itself. The chief academic officer in a school of nursing will no longer survive, nor will the school itself, with the old "seat of the pants" approach to administration. The administrator's repertoire must now include a firm grounding in administrative/organizational theory, financial management, organization development, marketing, public relations, and strategies for fund raising. In an era of cost control and limited resources, nursing is faced with balancing the need to cut costs and, therefore, programs on the one hand, and the need to generate more income on the other. The ability to prioritize and reallocate resources becomes paramount, and this ability depends in large part on the quantity and quality of information available for decision making. The presence of a comprehensive plan for program evaluation is vital to the generation of data necessary for systematic, goal-oriented decision making, and, in an era where competition is the hallmark, no strategic plan would be complete without a goal related to the development of a competitive marketing position for the school.

The administrative process is composed of four major elements— planning, organizing, leading, and evaluating. These elements must be seen as interrelated rather than separate if they are to facilitate the process, which is cyclical in nature. Planning is essentially the process of 1) setting goals; 2) defining those activities that need to be carried out in order to attain those goals; 3) determining how those activities can be most effectively organized, including the selection of individuals or groups responsible for producing the desired result; and 4) evaluating the organizational outcomes in relationship to the predetermined goals. Based on this assessment, original goals are redefined or modified. The element of organizing includes 1) the grouping of like activities, 2) the identification of formal power and organizational authority, and 3) the development of formal channels of communication. Overall organizing is the formal structuring of an institution or an activity. The element of planning must be organized, and the element of organizing must be planned, thus demonstrating the interrelationship of these two elements.

Leadership is perhaps the most complex of elements in the administrative process. There are probably as many definitions of leadership in the literature as there are authors who write on the subject. Perhaps the most that one can say about leadership is that it involves a thorough understanding of the concept of motivation, the ability to function within a complex communications network, and the selection of a leadership style that produces an effective interaction of the situation, the leader, and the follower. The age-old question of whether the administrator is a manager or a leader is explored by Abraham Zaleznik in an aticle in the *Harvard Business Review* (1977). Leaders, according to Zaleznik, are active instead of reactive; they shape ideas instead of responding to them. The net result of a leader's influence in altering moods, evoking images and expectations, and in establishing specific desires and objectives is to change the way people think about what is desirable, possible, and necessary. Leaders work to develop fresh approaches to longstanding problems and to open issues for new options. Such ideas, in fact, at times obsess the leader's mental life. To be effective, however, leaders need to project ideas into images that excite people and develop choices that give the projected images substance. Consequently, leaders create excitement in work. Leaders also tend to feel separate from their environment. They may work in organizations, but they never belong to them. Their sense of who they are does not depend on membership, work roles, or other social indicators of identity.

Evaluation keeps the administrative process energized and rational. It is a continuous, cyclical method of assessing both process (means) and outcome (ends). Leading and evaluating are integral to planning and organizing, and to each other. Thus, the administrative process and each of its elements are relative rather than constant, dynamic rather than static, and cyclical rather than one-dimensional. The process is goal oriented, and it is always a means to an end, never an end in itself. While the latter point may be obvious to most theoreticians, it is often lost in day-to-day organizational activity.

Everyone in an organization is involved in each of the elements of the administrative process to a greater or lesser degree, depending on one's role in the organization. Top-level administrators, for example, spend a greater proportion of their time in planning and organizing, while middle- and first-level administrators spend much of their time in leading and evaluating. However, it should be emphasized that everyone spends some proportion of his or her time in each of the administrative elements—this notion is critical to effective administration. More important to effectiveness is not just "doing things right" but "doing the right things." This is crucial if nursing is to survive the upheaval in the two major social systems of which it is such a part—the health care delivery system and the higher education system—that the administration of its programs reflects the trends in those social systems by planning and implementing strategies to keep nursing programs relevant. Thus, strategic planning becomes critical to effective administration.

PRINCIPLES AND APPROACHES TO STRATEGIC PLANNING

Kotler (1982) describes three types of nonprofit organizations: the responsive organization, the adaptive organization, and the entrepreneurial organization. According to Kotler, responsive organizations are those that "make every effort to sense, serve, and satisfy the needs and wants of its clients and publics within the constraints of its budget." Responsive organizations can be categorized into four levels of responsiveness: 1) unresponsive, 2) casually responsive, 3) highly responsive, and 4) fully responsive. It is altogether possible that nursing organizations, both practice- and education-oriented ones, fell into the first or second categories during their years of growth and expansion. In a seller's market, many organizations are bureaucratically operated, and means become ends in themselves. Thus, the institution does not involve itself at all in determining consumer needs and wants, or it restricts itself to making these determinations but does not follow through by making relevant organizational changes. Given the current buyer's market for nursing services and nursing education, most health care organizations and schools of nursing fall into the third, or highly responsive, category. These groups seek ways to improve consumer services and train their personnel to be consumer-oriented. Some institutions are moving toward becoming fully responsive by creating means for consumers to participate actively in the organization's affairs. Hospital boards and advisory committees include consumers, and school of nursing committees have long included students and nurses engaged in nursing practice, thus giving them a voice in institutional governance.

An adaptive organization is "one that operates systems for monitoring and interpreting important environmental changes and shows a readiness to revise its mission, objectives, strategies, organization, and systems to be maximally aligned with its opportunities" (Kotler, 1982, p. 76). Factors that affect the organization's capacity to change include size (smaller organizations are usually more adaptive than larger organizations), funds (organizations with larger financial resources are more adaptive than organizations with fewer financial resources), leadership (an organization led by someone who is more interested in making it work than in preserving its form is likely to be more adaptive), and constraints (private, profit-oriented, internally controlled organizations are more adaptive than highly regulated, nonprofit, and public organizations).

An entrepreneurial organization is one with a high motivation and the capability to identify new opportunities and convert them into successful businesses. Temporary service agencies owned and managed by nurses, nurses practicing directly with an elderly community population, and nurses providing home care services for patients with AIDS are all examples of successful entrepreneurial ventures. Innovative faculty practice plans and marketing educational products are entrepreneurial ventures in some schools of nursing. While entrepreneurial organizations go one step further than a responsive or adaptive organization, they grow out of an organization's interaction with its environment; thus, they develop frequently as a result of the adaptive organization's strategic plan.

Strategic planning, as a management tool, is directed toward improving organizational performance. Strategic planning is "the managerial process of developing and maintaining a strategic fit between the organization's goals and resources and its changing marketing opportunities" (Kotler, 1982, p. 83). Morrison and Cope (1985), in comparing strategic planning to long-range planning, state that strategic planning is usually characterized as "outside-in" planning and places emphasis on the environment. It also pulls together soft and hard data to arrive at major directional decisions. Keller (1983) indicates that strategic planning cannot be neatly defined, but he indicates that, among other things, it is 1) not the production of a blueprint, but rather a process of getting key people thinking innovatively with the future in mind; 2) not a set of platitudes, but rather the formulation of succinctly stated operational aims; 3) not a collection of departmental plans, compiled and edited, but rather a plan for the whole institution in relation to its long-term stature and excellence; 4) not a substitution of numbers for important intangibles, but rather the introduction of these to sharpen judgments, analyses, and decisions; and 5) not an attempt to outwit the future, but rather an effort to make this year's decisions more intelligent by looking toward the probable future and coupling decisions to an overall institutional strategy. Strategic decisions are based on the best evidence available about the unpredictable future.

Keller (1983, pp. 143–150) describes six features that characterize strategic planning:

1. Strategic decision making means that an organization and its leaders are proactive, rather than reactive, in determining its place in history.
2. Strategic planning looks outward and is focused on keeping the institution in step with the changing environment.
3. Strategy making is competitive, recognizing that health care and higher education are subject to economic market conditions and to increasingly strong competition.
4. Strategic planning is action-oriented, concentrating on decisions, not on documented plans, analyses, forecasts, and goals.
5. Strategy making is a blend of rational and economic analysis, political maneuvering, and psychological interplay. It is participatory and highly tolerant of controversy. Dissent is permitted; sabotage is not. The chief administrative officer is the final arbiter, the ultimate shaper of strategy.
6. Strategic planning concentrates on the fate of the institution above everything else. Therefore, it should be the first priority of top-level administrators.

Even though the necessity for strategic planning is well documented in both the health care industry and in higher education, there is frequently a gap between the ideal and the real. Nonprofit organizations, in particular, have not been known for their strong bent toward strategic planning. Several explanations for "not getting around to it" exist. Among these are the following:

1. Crisis-oriented management that focuses on "putting out fires" instead of focusing on developing a reasonable "fire proof" environment.
2. Overemphasis on individuality that creates vested interests that override the common good of the institution.

3. Fear of organizational change and the perhaps undesirable side effects of an otherwise desirable plan.

4. Fear of making mistakes because of the uncertainty of dealing with a rapidly changing environment.

5. Fear of the personal threat implied by the power and politics of the process.

6. Lack of leadership, preparation, vision, or interest.

Even when organizations do get around to strategic planning, they may find that they are organized for the work of the past and not of the future. With regard to the present, prospective planners often see each other as being out of step with the world when the problem is that none of them has an accurate perception of the world. Keller points out in his book, *Academic Strategy*, that it is difficult to convince faculties that higher education is big business. Until the advent of the PPS, it was equally difficult to sell that notion to the health care industry. Both systems have been reluctant to change even in response to market demands, creating the potentially disastrous situation that administrators can't act, and faculties and health care providers won't act. Faculties and nurses in the practice arena must be willing and able to assume the role of guiding the institution's development or concede to others the right to do so.

Strategic planning emphasizes the future direction of an institution. Successful institutions have a vision of the future and a strategy for realizing that vision. To help ensure success, not only strategic planning but also strategic thinking and management must be in place. According to Green and Monical (1985),

> Strategic planning poses four fundamental questions: Where have we been and where are we now? Where will we be in the future by following our present course? Where do we want to be? How will we get there? The successful performance of an organization relates directly to effective planning, decision making, and execution. An organization that determines where it plans to go, what it plans to do, and how it plans to do it, can make better decisions, more effectively manage resources and operations, and adjust more readily to change. (p. 49)

The ability to plan, think, and manage strategically, including the ability to prioritize and reallocate resources, becomes paramount in an era of cost control and limited resources. This ability depends in large part on the quantity and quality of information available for decision making. In an educational institution, for example, an ongoing program of institutional research should generate such information as the following: 1) projections of enrollment results based upon new marketing procedures that reduce error between projected and actual enrollment; 2) program reviews of academic offerings that show the cost-effectiveness of each program and department; 3) measures of student attitude and performance to determine the holding influence of the institution; 4) marketing and accounting strategies to determine whether support services such as the media center, research center, and student services are cost-effective; 5) facility utilization results to gauge the needed investment in renovation and maintenance; 6) plans for generating dollars to balance the budget and provide needed funding for new equipment and maintenance when there are not enough funds to cover such expenditures; and 7) fund-raising strategies related to specific operational goals, endowment, or capital campaign needs (Ringle & Saveckas, 1983). Good planning in both nursing practice and nursing education requires sound, data-based decision making, program evaluation, and institutional research. Outcome measurement is a vital component of each.

ORGANIZING FOR STRATEGIC PLANNING

In spite of the fact that there are many advocates of "bottom-up," as opposed to "top-down," planning, organizations differ tremendously. Because there are different kinds of institutions, there need to be different kinds of strategic-planning processes. Some observers would argue in favor of "top-down" planning based on the mode of administration that indicates that the higher one's role is in the organizational structure, the greater is the proportion of one's time spent in planning. The process needs to be tailored to the institutional situation. However, there are some basic tenets to keep in mind when one is mobilizing for strategic planning. "Every organization needs to have a forcible champion of good management and planning," according to Keller (1983, p. 165). In nursing practice, it should be the vice president for nursing or chief administrative officer of the nursing department. In schools of nursing, it should be the dean or chief administrative officer of the nursing education unit. Keller (1983, p. 166) states, "More efforts at improvement and better planning collapse because of the lack of consistent advocacy by the top leadership and persistent monitoring of divisional plans than for any other reason." Needless to say, chief administrative officers of nursing units need to understand their own role in the organization and how they relate to others, both inside and outside their own institution. They need second-level administrators to whom they delegate major program responsibility and whom they hold accountable for productivity in that program. Only then can moving the institution forward in a strategic manner become the administrator's top priority. When this occurs, emphasis is placed on "doing the right things" rather than "doing things right." Green and Monical (1985, p. 54) point out that "if the overall strategy of an organization is correct, any number of tactical errors can be made without significantly hurting the organization. However, if the overall strategy is wrong, the organization will fail in its efforts no matter how many tactical efforts are right." Administrators who function successfully in a decentralized structure know how to focus on doing things right.

Caruthers (1981, pp. 23–24) indicates that several conditions for successful planning relate to organization. Of these, he states that "leadership and staffing requirements are probably the most important." Staff support is essential, not only for data collection and analysis, but also to provide input on the history, environment, and current operations of the institution.

Where strategic planning is concerned, participation can be the key to better decisions and successful implementation. Each participant needs the technical expertise to address the issues at hand. Certainly, those who will be affected by planning decisions need to be represented. The key word here is *represented*, since not everyone in the organization can participate *directly* in strategic planning. Sometimes, the time frame for completing activity and scheduling concerns determines the approach to planning. For example, if there are no time constraints, and it is particularly important to establish a broad base of support, the "bottom-up" approach to planning might be better than the more efficient "top-down" approach. One "advantage of strategic planning is that it often is involved simultaneously in the use of top-down, bottom-up, and team approaches to planning, thus enhancing the value of communication within the organization" (Green & Monical, 1985, p. 49). There is no right or wrong way to organize for strategic planning. A structure should be designed that takes into consideration the organization's readiness as well as its style and other needs.

Hipps (1982, pp. 115–130) describes a generalized model for change that can be used as the basis for the strategic-planning process. He lists eight elements that he believes essential to any institution attempting to effect organizational change: 1) definition of organizational mission, 2) top-administrative support, 3) leadership development, 4) comprehensive change programs, 5) participation, 6) emphasis on communication, 7) emphasis on process, and 8) merging of individual and institutional goals. While these elements are not meant to provide a "blueprint" for strategic planning, the following chapter will illustrate their utility in the strategic-planning process.

REFERENCES

Caruthers, J. K. (1981). Strategic master plans. In N. L. Poulton (Ed.), *Evaluation of management and planning systems* (pp. 23–24). New Directions for Institutional Research Series. San Francisco: Jossey-Bass.

Fagin, C. M. (1982, December). The economic value of nursing research. *American Journal of Nursing, 82*(12), 1840.

Green, J. L., & Monical, D. G. (1985, December). Resource allocation in a decentralized environment. In D. J. Berg & G. Skogley (Eds.), *Making the budget process work* (pp. 49, 54). New Dimensions for Higher Education, No. 52. San Francisco: Jossey-Bass.

Hipps, G. M. (1982). Summary and conclusions. In G. Melvin Hipps (Ed.), *Effective planned change strategies. New directions for institutional research series* (pp. 115–130). San Francisco: Jossey-Bass.

Keller, G. (1983). *Academic strategy.* Baltimore: The Johns Hopkins University Press.

Kotler, P. (1982). *Marketing for non-profit organizations.* Englewood Cliffs, NJ: Prentice-Hall, Inc.

Morrison, J. L., & Cope, R. G. (1985). Future research techniques in strategic planning: A simulation. *Planning for Higher Education, 13*(2), 5–9.

National League for Nursing. (1984, April 12). Testimony on Title VIII, Public Health Service Act, Submitted by National League for Nursing to the Energy and Commerce Subcommittee on Health and the Environment. New York: National League for Nursing.

Ringle, P. M., & Saveckas, M. L. (1983). Administrative leadership. *Journal of Higher Education*, 649–661.

Zaleznik, A. (1977, May–June). Managers and leaders: Are they different? *Harvard Business Review*, 67–78.

2

Implementing Strategic Planning

Nan B. Hechenberger

This chapter utilizes the case study approach to demonstrate the implementation of the strategic-planning process. Included are illustrations of selected strategies and techniques for successful planning, organizational analysis and formulation of long-range goals, plan development, and plan implementation and control. What is described is a process of organization development spanning a 10-year period (1978–1988) in a large, publicly supported school of nursing situated in an academic health center in a metropolitan area on the East Coast of the United States. Even though the organization exemplified in this presentation is a large, complex part of a major research university, the planning process described is applicable to smaller, less-complex educational settings as well as in nursing practice settings.

This administrative odyssey actually began when the present dean of the school of nursing was a candidate for that position. The search committee required each of the four finalists for the position of dean to present a colloquium for faculty and students of the school of nursing. This colloquium was to address issues and trends in higher education, nursing education, and nursing; future directions for the school of nursing; and administrative style.

In discussing issues and trends in higher education, the dean candidate's emphasis was on the fact that, in 1978, higher education was in financial depression, and the associated diminution of public confidence in institutions of higher education had been accompanied by an increasing number of external controls by federal and state regulatory agencies and by changes in internal priorities. Another implication of limited resources is that academic planning must include review of existing programs for the dual purposes of developing quality programs and the termination of ineffective and unproductive programs. The implication that programs would be terminated as well as developed was something that institutions had generally been unwilling to face. It was important to bear these issues in mind as they shaped the setting in which the dean of a school of nursing would function.

The colloquium paper went on to describe changes in the field of health (and, therefore, in nursing and nursing education) and in public expectations of health professions, which, combined, caused a major change in the structure of nursing schools, their relationships to other health sciences schools, the rest of the university, and society in general. These changes had put enormous stress on the administrative structure of nursing schools and on those responsible for the administration of these institutions. In addition, the paper spoke to the triple mission of the university, the preparation and utilization of professional nurses, and the establishment of a collegial relationship with nursing service and other health disciplines.

The dean candidate probed roles and relationships of the dean as they pertain to the organizational functions of academic, faculty, and student affairs, development (including alumni, public, and governmental relations), and finances. These comments were predicated on the assumption that the process of administration requires the dean to spend some proportion of his or her time in each of the organizational processes: planning, organizing, leading, and evaluating. The candidate stated that the dean, particularly in a large, complex organization with several educational programs, needs to spend considerably more time on activities related to planning and organizing than on those related to leadership and evaluation. She stated, "This implies that the dean has to be willing and able to 'let go'—to delegate responsibility and authority for specific functions and programs and to hold the appropriate persons accountable." She elaborated, "For example, I believe that the development and articulation of the philosophy, goals, and objectives of the school are primarily the prerogative of the faculty, but that these need to be realistically stated within the boundary of local, state, and regional planning patterns and within guidelines dictated by both the actual and potential resources of the school in terms of faculty, facilities, and finances. To set unrealistic goals is to build in failure and frustration at the outset" (Hechenberger, 1981, p. 23). She indicated that in addition to the ability to set organizational goals, it is important to establish and maintain good, purposeful interpersonal relationships both inside and outside the school if the dean is to be successful. In addition, she pointed out that the dean is responsible for providing leadership in academic, faculty, and student affairs and for providing a mechanism for ongoing evaluation and development of both personnel and programs.

During the colloquium, the candidate indicated that her initial priority would be to implement an organization-wide development program. This program would involve a systematic survey of the organizational climate as perceived by faculty, staff, and students; sharing the results of this survey with faculty, staff, and students; mutual prioritization of problems to be solved; and the designing of strategies to deal with these problems. In April 1978, the candidate envisioned a need for some version of team building, management by objectives, and structural changes beginning at top organizational levels and filtering down. Implicit in this priority is the fact that institutional performance is at risk unless the development of its administrators is viewed as a top priority. The candidate's second priority was related to the evaluation, upgrading, and expansion of the existing programs. In this regard, she gave special attention to the further development and implementation of the doctoral program; expansion of the continuing education program and the outreach program; decentralization of the faculty orientation and development program; and the implementation of evening, summer, and weekend classes. Her third priority was the decentralization of the budget, envisioning, at first, decentralization to the levels of the primary units in the school (i.e., the undergraduate, graduate, and continuing education programs) with the associate deans and the director of continuing education responsible for budget planning and administration within their own units. Further decentralization would be determined by the organizational structure at the time of decentralization.

When this candidate became the dean of the school of nursing in October 1978, she met with the faculty and reiterated her priorities for the school. She also reiterated her previous comments on the constraints of limited financial resources and increasing external regulation. She spoke of her determination to move the school forward in a logical and organized manner but also noted that thought is a prelude and not an alternative to action. As Will Rogers once said, "Even if you're on the right track, you'll get run over if you just sit there."

At this point, the organization was large and complex. There were approximately 1,200 students enrolled in its undergraduate and graduate programs, and there were approximately 160 faculty members.

The baccalaureate program for registered nurses and selected areas of concentration in the master's program were offered in two rural areas of the state in addition to being offered at the city campus. The master's program was quite diverse, offering 10 areas of concentration. Over 100 agencies were utilized to provide clinical experiences for students. Figure 1 is an organization chart depicting the organizational structure of the school of nursing as it existed in 1978.

During the prior 10 years, the school had undergone rapid growth and experienced a high rate of turnover at the associate dean level. Since associate deans were essentially program heads for undergraduate and graduate programs, the impact of this turnover reverberated throughout these academic programs. In addition, there had been personnel changes in every position in the university that directly impacted on faculty (i.e., there was a new president of the university, a new vice president for academic affairs, a new chancellor of the Academic Health Center, and a new dean of the School of Nursing). Without exception, the leadership style of each of these individuals was substantially different from the style of his or her predecessor. The school of nursing was ready for internal change.

"Organizational Development (OD) is a response to change, a complex educational strategy intended to change the beliefs, attitudes, values, and structure of organizations so that they can better adapt to new technologies, markets, and challenges, and the dizzying rate of change itself," according to Bennis (1969, p. 2). In essence, it is an educational strategy adopted to bring about a planned organizational change. Although business and industry had been consciously applying OD strategies to their operations for approximately 25 years, the concept in 1978 was relatively new in institutions of higher education.

In order to make data-based decisions relevant to what kind of changes were necessary, an organizational assessment of "problem areas" was undertaken using the Woodcock Blockage Questionnaire (Francis & Woodcock, 1975). Essentially, the questionnaire elicits data relevant to blocks to the effective use of people in an organization, decreasing the effectiveness of the system as a whole. Use of this instrument, it should be noted, elicits only negative data related to "problem areas." It does not elicit positive data related to organizational strengths. Blockage areas identified by the questionnaire are 1) inadequate recruitment and selection, 2) confused organizational structure, 3) inadequate control, 4) poor training, 5) low motivation, 6) low creativity, 7) poor teamwork, 8) inappropriate management philosophy, 9) lack of succession planning and management, 10) unclear aims, and 11) unfair rewards. The questionnaire as modified is included in the appendix.

Figure 1
School of Nursing Organization Chart (1978)

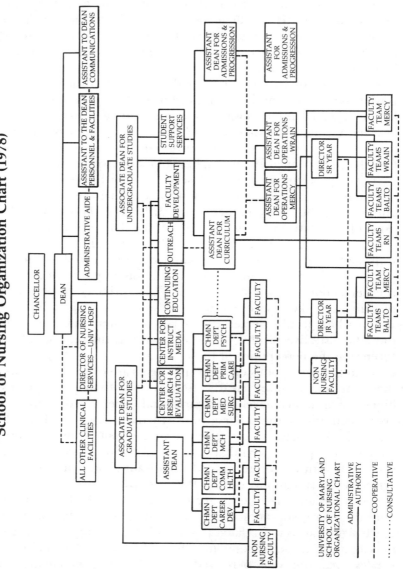

UNIVERSITY OF MARYLAND
SCHOOL OF NURSING
ORGANIZATIONAL CHART

ADMINISTRATIVE
AUTHORITY

-------- COOPERATIVE

············· CONSULTATIVE

The questionnaire was administered to all faculty and staff in the school of nursing, with a 58 percent response rate. Data were analyzed in relation to the following variables: 1) employment status (faculty or staff), 2) faculty rank, 3) program (undergraduate, graduate, continuing education), 4) graduate department, 5) primary responsibility (teaching or administration), 6) tenure status, 7) length of employment, and 8) educational background. An item analysis (10 items for each blockage area) was also done.

An analysis of the data indicated that "poor teamwork" was perceived as a major problem, with confused organizational structure, low motivation, unfair rewards, low creativity, and inadequate control also having high blockage scores. The blockage area perceived to be the least problematic was "inappropriate management philosophy." Clearly, the group with the highest blockage scores (indicating more perceived problem areas) was the secretarial staff. In six blockage areas (recruitment, control, training, motivation, management philosophy, and rewards), there were significant differences between the perceptions of the staff and those of the faculty. There were no significant differences in the perceptions of faculty when compared according to rank and tenure status. "Poor teamwork" was ranked as the primary problem area across faculty ranks. There was a significant difference in the perceptions of faculty members whose primary responsibility was teaching and those whose primary responsibility was administration, with teaching faculty perceiving the reward system as more unfair than did administrative faculty. This, however, was the only significant difference in the perceptions of these two groups.

When the perceptions of the respondents are compared according to their educational level, clearly, the group with high school as their highest educational level (secretarial staff) perceived more blockage areas than any of the other groups. In fact, they scored significantly higher in four areas (recruitment, training, motivation, inappropriate management philosophy) than did any of the other groups. Those respondents with doctorates scored significantly lower in regard to perceived rewards than any of the other groups.

It was obvious that the longer the respondent had been in the system, the more blockages were perceived. The only blockage score to reach significance was related to succession planning and management development; those respondents who had been employed in the school for less than one year perceived this to be less problematic than did those who had been in the school longer. This was congruent with the fact that tenured faculty perceived more blockages overall than did nontenured employees.

There were no significant differences in the perceptions of faculty when compared across graduate departments. Poor teamwork was again perceived as the leading problem. There were no significant differences, with one exception, in the perceptions of faculty in the undergraduate, graduate, and continuing education programs. Graduate faculty scored significantly lower than the other two groups with regard to their perception of the reward system. This coincided with the perceptions of faculty members with doctorates.

The results of the survey were reported to the faculty (survey feedback is a diagnostic technique frequently utilized in OD efforts), and plans were made to address the problems identified in the survey via a year-long management development program for academic administrators in the school of nursing. Participants included the dean, the associate and assistant deans, chairs in the undergraduate and graduate program, and directors of support units in the school of nursing. According to Beckhard (1969), there is a basic difference between management development and organization development. Management development might be viewed as "manager development," in that the target is the development, improvement, or assessment of the individual manager. Organization development includes management development efforts, but it is primarily focused on improving the systems that make up the total organization. As part of the overall organization development plan for the school of nursing, a series of three workshops for academic administrators was planned. These were held off-campus, with an overnight stay required. The dean of a large university school of education served as workshop leader and consultant for the year. Each workshop was planned collaboratively by the dean of the school of nursing, the director of continuing education and faculty development, and the workshop leader/consultant. It should be noted that very few of the members of the academic-administrator group had formal educational preparation in administration.

During the first session, the role of the academic administrator, both in general and from the perspectives of supervisors and of subordinates, was explored on the assumption that one responsibility of the academic administrator is to create a healthy organizational climate. The characteristics of a healthy academic climate were also explored. The administrators then compared perceptions of their own organizational climate (based on responses by faculty and staff to the Woodcock Blockage Questionnaire) with the characteristics of a healthy organization. The purpose of making this comparison was to 1) identify gaps between the academic environment in the school of nursing and the healthy academic environment, 2) identify the effects of these disparities in achieving the mission of the school, 3) identify what must be done to make the school of nursing environment more congruent with the healthy model, and 4) identify priorities for action.

Problems for action were prioritized based on the percentage of people in the overall sample who marked each item as a problem, and strategies for coping with problem areas were developed by the academic administrators for the undergraduate, graduate, and continuing education programs, as well as for academic services. These strategies were to be implemented in the school of nursing during the period between October 1979 and February 1980. At the second workshop in February, problems encountered in strategy implementation were identified with particular emphasis on process-related problems. Much of the session was devoted to the concept of leadership. Strategies related to improving interpersonal and leadership skills were developed and implemented in the work setting.

Following assessment of the organizational climate and implementation of administrative strategies to cope with areas identified as problematic, the Woodcock Blockage Questionnaire was administered for a second time, with a 61 percent response rate. Analysis of the results indicated a significant reduction in each of the perceived blockage areas. In addition to strategy evaluation, the third administrative development session was used to identify priorities for the 1980–1981 program. It is important to note that these sessions included more than an administrative development objective, in that there was actual follow-up and strategy implementation between sessions in order to evaluate and reevaluate progress. The intention was that these workshops would give the academic administrators a better understanding of their organizational roles, strengthen their leadership skills, and provide them with some sense of excitement about meeting the challenges facing them.

Other outcomes of the assessment of the organizational climate included a reorganization of the administrative and governance structure in the school of nursing, resulting in the reduction of structure levels from six to three, the reshuffling and merger of 10 major areas of concentration at the master's level (reducing the number of graduate departments from six to three), and a change in the bylaws of the school of nursing that halved the number of faculty committees from 12 to six. Figure 2 shows the new administrative structure in the school of nursing. In addition, a Master Plan for Program Evaluation (University of Maryland School of Nursing, 1982) and a Prescriptive Plan for Faculty Assignment, Evaluation, and Development (University of Maryland School of Nursing, 1982) were developed.

Figure 2
School of Nursing Organization Chart (1980)

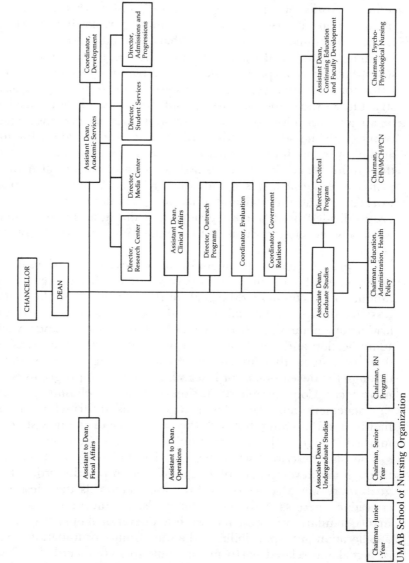

CHANCELLOR

DEAN

Assistant to Dean, Fiscal Affairs

Assistant to Dean, Operations

Coordinator, Development

Assistant Dean, Academic Services

Director, Research Center

Director, Media Center

Director, Student Services

Director, Admissions and Progressions

Assistant Dean, Clinical Affairs

Director, Outreach Programs

Coordinator, Evaluation

Coordinator, Government Relations

Associate Dean, Undergraduate Studies

Chairman, Junior -Year

Chairman, Senior Year

Chairman, RN Program

Associate Dean, Graduate Studies

Director, Doctoral Program

Chairman, Education, Administration, Health Policy

Chairman, CHN/MCH/PCN

Assistant Dean, Continuing Education and Faculty Development

Chairman, Psycho-Physiological Nursing

UMAB School of Nursing Organization

By 1983, there was a decided readiness within the school of nursing for strategic planning. Dr. George Keller, author of *Academic Strategy: The Management Revolution in American Higher Education* (1983), presented a workshop on strategic planning and marketing for the academic administrators in the school of nursing. Following the workshop, the administrative group decided that it would serve as the primary planning group, with the addition of the coordinator for evaluation, who would serve as primary staff to the planning project. The coordinator for evaluation reports directly to the dean in the organizational structure of the school of nursing, but the position is not considered to be an administrative one; the coordinator does not meet as a matter of course with the administrative group. The vice president for nursing at the university hospital participated as an external representative to the group. While she serves as assistant dean for Clinical Affairs, her primary responsibility is in nursing practice. Although the plan was worked out at the day-and-a-half-long administrative retreats, the group divided itself into subgroups and did a substantial amount of work between these sessions. It took almost one year for the plan to develop.

The plan includes a statement of mission, which identifies the school as an integral part of a university academic health center, with a unique role in combining the goals of the university and those of a professional discipline. The mission of the school of nursing is to provide leadership in nursing through scholarship, research, and evaluation. Identification and development of areas of practice and nursing care delivery systems that anticipate and are responsive to societal needs through the development of research and teaching programs is the primary focus. Considerable discussion over the development of the mission statement took place. The primary focus of this school historically had been on teaching, but with the acceptance of the new statement, a marked change in the organization's norms was mandated.

The plan described what the school would have by the year 1990, through the development of 11 goals listed in priority order. For each goal, there was a series of performance standards that described the conditions necessary to meet the goals. Furthermore, each performance standard was broken down into operational objectives, each with an allocation of responsibility and a time frame for initiation. Examples of a goal and related performance standards are included in Table 1.

The goal with the highest priority rating shown in Table 1 is "A climate and environment that facilitates and supports faculty research and scholarship activities." The high-priority rating for this goal

Table 1
Example of Goal and Related Performance Standards

Goal	Performance Standards
By the year 1990, the school of nursing will have:	It will be necessary for the following conditions to exist to justify that the school of nursing goals have been met:
1. A climate and environment that facilitates and supports faculty research and scholarship activities	1. The number of faculty on self-supporting research grants has increased 2. Private offices have been provided for all senior faculty 3. Research laboratories for bench research have been made accessible 4. Collaborative working relationships between clinical agency personnel and faculty conducting research projects have been established 5. Funded interdisciplinary research has been undertaken 6. Space and the number of faculty in the research center have increased 7. Documented evidence has been obtained to justify that the location of units and the assignment of space facilitate research 8. Appropriate equipment for research activities has been made readily accessible and available to faculty (i.e., hardware, computer terminals, word processors, and software) 9. The number of funded research projects has increased 10. On the average, the equivalent of 20% of the total salaries of the senior faculty has been secured from external funding 11. The number of publications in juried journals has increased 12. Research support systems have been strengthened and expanded (e.g., support staff, measurement file) 13. Funds and research assistants available for the support of preliminary (pilot) studies have increased 14. Research productivity has been reflected in appointments, promotions, and tenure and merit increase decisions 15. The number of individuals engaged in postdoctoral study has increased

seemed to be appropriate for a school of nursing whose parent institution is a major research university. Examples of performance standards for this goal include the following: 1) the number of faculty on self-supporting research grants has increased, 2) appropriate equipment for research activities has been made readily accessible and available to faculty, and 3) on the average, the equivalent of 20 percent of the total salaries of senior faculty has been secured from external funding. There is a total of 15 performance standards for this goal, with 47 operational objectives involving 160 people over a period of six years in goal implementation. Table 2 illustrates some of the operational objectives needed to meet the performance standards for this goal. Table 3 illustrates the responsibilities and time frame for implementing operational objectives.

The second-highest priority was assigned to the goal "Programs are planned and decisions made that are justified on the basis of evaluation data from a variety of sources." Among the performance standards developed for this goal are that 1) the Master Plan for Evaluation and a marketing analysis have been implemented, and 2) organizational and program priorities, including those within programs, have been established. In order to meet the latter standard, criteria were developed to prioritize the 18 program offerings at the master's level. Five criteria were related to faculty (e.g., "Programs given priority status are pro-

Table 2
Example of Goal and Selected Operational Objectives

Goal	Operational Objectives
A climate and environment that facilitates and supports faculty research and scholarship activities	1. Secure additional external funds to support preliminary (pilot) studies 2. Place emphasis on research productivity in actions related to appointment, promotion, and tenure and merit increase decisions 3. Provide workshops and consultations on publishing scholarly papers for faculty and students 4. Acquire for each department a computer terminal and a word processor 5. Increase research space to include psychosocial labs, data processing rooms, interviewing rooms, and physiological monitoring equipment 6. Seek funding for programs of postdoctoral study

Table 3
Example of Selected Operational Objectives, Responsibility, and Time Frame for Initiation

Operational Objective	Responsibility	Time Frame for Initiation
1. Secure additional external funds to support preliminary studies	Dean, chairs, individual faculty	May 1983
2. Place emphasis on research productivity in actions related to appointment, promotion, and tenure and merit increase decisions	Academic administrators	May 1983
3. Provide workshops and consultations on publishing scholarly papers for faculty and students	Assistant dean for continuing education; director, research center; departments	June 1984
4. Acquire for each department a computer terminal and a word processor	Assistant dean for academic services	January 1985
5. Increase research space to include psychosocial labs, data processing and interviewing rooms, and physiological monitoring equipment	Dean	June 1986
6. Seek funding for programs of postdoctoral study	Associate dean for graduate studies	June 1987

vided by outstanding faculty whose research and publications make a unique contribution to the profession"), seven criteria were related to students (e.g., "Programs of given priority status are those that attract large numbers of highly qualified and diverse applicants"), 10 criteria were related to the program itself (e.g., "Programs given priority status are those that are of higher quality as evidenced by evaluation data than are the same or similar programs offered by competitors"), two criteria were related to resources (e.g., "Programs given priority status are those that the school of nursing has unique and/or outstanding specific resources to offer that are not generally available elsewhere"), and nine criteria were related to cost (e.g., "Programs given priority status are those that can justify their cost on the basis of relevance, need, and demand for graduates").

For each criterion, it was necessary to consider the answers to certain questions about existing and proposed programs in order to establish the relative importance of each, in regard to information gleaned from data. In addition, it was necessary to consider what was available and what needed to be established via the Master Plan for Evaluation, marketing analyses, and other sources in order to answer each question. Table 4 illustrates selected criteria, suggested questions, and potential sources for each question. Faculty were asked to use professional judgment in rating the extent to which each criterion was achieved within the particular specialty program. They were asked to rate the extent of achievement of the current program on each criterion on a scale of 1 (not at all) through 9 (completely); they were also requested to use available data and examples to provide the rationale for their judgment.

The academic administrator responsible for each program presented the data to all of the school of nursing academic administrators at one of the administrative retreats. Following these presentations and a discussion, a Delphi technique (Waltz, Strickland, & Lenz, 1984, pp. 281–285) was employed in an attempt to obtain data that reflected the majority view of the academic administrators about what program(s) should be eliminated and given priority in the reallocation of scarce resources. Although the ultimate decision-making responsibility rested with the school of nursing executive committee (dean, associate deans, and assistant deans), the collective view of the academic administrators was seen as important input into the process.

Each member of the academic administrators' group was asked by mail to complete a series of rankings of the specialty tracks in the master's program. Once the completed rankings were returned by mail to the dean's office and anaylzed by staff in the office of evaluation, responses were tabulated and summarized. Since the interest was in majority views, frequency distributions and the mode served as a basis for the decision regarding when the majority view was reflected in the data. A summary of the findings from the first series of rankings was returned to the group by mail. Each individual in the group was asked to consider the information in the summary and to then complete and return a second series of rankings. In order to preserve anonymity, each individual was asked to keep a copy of his own completed rankings so that they could readily be compared with the summary data provided at the time of the second series of rankings. The process was terminated at the completion of the third series of rankings, when the resulting data clearly reflected a majority view of the group.

The specialty tracks were ranked in two ways: for elimination from the master's program (from 1 [first to be eliminated] to 18 [last to be eliminated]) and for priority when master's program resources are reallocated (from 1 [first priority] to 18 [last priority]). When the data

Table 4
Selected Criteria and Management Data Needs
for the Determination of Program Priorities

Criteria: Programs given priority status are provided by outstanding faculty whose research and publications make a unique contribution to the profession

Questions	Potential data sources
Is a high level of scholarly productivity maintained by faculty?	1. Comparison of academic rank among four health profession schools 2. Ongoing faculty research 3. Criteria for appointments, promotion, tenure
What types of leadership do faculty provide in regard to research and publication in the profession of nursing?	1. Faculty vitae

Criteria: Programs given priority status are those that attract large numbers of highly qualified and diverse applicants

What efforts are undertaken by the program to actively recruit highly qualified and diversified applicants?	1. Marketing analysis: organizational analysis phase
Is the process by which students are recruited, reviewed, and selected for admission to the program effective and efficient?	1. Master Plan for Program Evaluation 2. Institutional Research Data

Criteria: Programs given priority status are those that are of higher quality as evidenced by evaluation data than are the same or similar programs offered by competitors

What is known of the quality of the same or similar programs offered by competitors?	1. Marketing analysis: competitive phase
What do we know of students' general academic potential before admission?	1. Master Plan for Program Evaluation 2. GPA, GRE, MAT Scores

Criteria: Programs given priority status are those that the school of nursing has unique and/or outstanding specific resources to offer that are not generally available elsewhere

Is the School of Nursing the only place where a given specific resource is available?	1. Marketing analysis: competitive and organizational phases
What resources not currently utilized does the School of Nursing have access to that competitors do not?	1. Marketing analysis 2. Organizational analysis

Criteria: Programs given priority status are those that can justify their cost on the basis of relevance, need, and demand for graduates

What is the demand for graduates of the program? Are graduates employed in the areas for which they were prepared?	1. Marketing analysis: Market analysis phase 2. Master Plan for Program Evaluation
Is there evidence that the program is relevant, unique, and/or competitive enough to justify the current costs?	1. Marketing analysis: competitive phase

were analyzed, the first three specialty tracks targeted for elimination from the master's program were the last three targeted for reallocation, and the first three specialty tracks targeted for reallocation were the last three targeted for elimination.

The original strategic plan was developed as a 1983–1990 plan. In 1986, the plan was evaluated and revised. Goals were reprioritized, and accomplishments toward the goals and objectives were assessed. For example, one of the operational objectives listed for the goal, "A climate and environment that facilitates and supports faculty research and scholarship activities" was "secure additional external funds to support preliminary (pilot) studies" (see Table 2). In the revised planning document, listed under "accomplishments toward goals and objectives" is the statement, "Funds to support preliminary studies have been made available via the DRIF (Designated Research Initiative Fund) funds (a total of 14 projects supported last year)."

In addition, activities related to the accomplishment of goals and objectives were developed for fiscal year 1988, and a five-year activity plan for fiscal years 1989–1993 was developed. Constraints/resources needed were included in the plan for each goal, reflecting a change in the environment for nursing education. The goal that in 1983 had been prioritized as first moved down to second. In 1986, the goal with the highest priority rating was "Adequate funding from private and public sources to support the delivery of high quality programs." This goal had been prioritized as third in the original strategic plan.

In an era where "competition" is the hallmark, no strategic plan would be complete without a goal related to "developing a competitive marketing position locally, regionally, and nationally among schools of nursing." Subsequently, a schoolwide marketing plan that includes a statement of the current market position, long- and short-range marketing objectives and goals, criteria for measurement of goal achievement, a statement of strategies for the school of nursing, an action plan designed to achieve the strategies, and a budget was developed. Nursing service personnel need to be involved intimately with the school in the development of a marketing plan. The vice president for nursing at the university hospital was involved throughout the strategic planning process. The notion of maintaining collaborative relationships with a variety of clinical agencies in order to promote greater effectiveness and efficiency in the use of nursing resources in the care of patients, education of nurses, and the conduct of research and evaluation studies is imperative.

This case study is an illustration of the four phases of strategic planning: 1) environmental scanning and analysis, 2) institutional mission and goals, 3) performance standards and strategies, and 4) action plan and priorities. The strategic planning process in this particular school of nursing remains viable because the master plan is monitored through the matching of its implementation schedule and the completion of specific tasks. It has been necessary to adjust schedules and to change priorities based on the realities of both the external and internal environments for the school of nursing, but this is part of the dynamic process of strategic planning. In this instance, the plan is a means to a end, not an end in itself. It is an ongoing, decision-making model in which the process is more important than the product.

REFERENCES

Beckhard, R. (1969). *Organization development: Strategies and models* (pp. 20–22). Reading, MA: Addison-Wesley.

Bennis, W. G. (1969). *Organization development: Its nature, origins, and prospects* (p. 2). Reading, MA: Addison-Wesley.

Francis, D., & Woodcock, M. (1975). *People at work: A practical guide to organizational change*. La Jolla, CA: University Associates, Inc.

Hechenberger, N. B. (1981). The dean as administrator. In *Executive development series I: "Have you ever thought of being a dean?"*, AACN, *1*, 20–29.

Keller, G. (1983). *Academic strategy*. Baltimore: Johns Hopkins University Press.

University of Maryland School of Nursing. (1982). *Master plan for program evaluation*. Baltimore: University of Maryland School of Nursing.

University of Maryland School of Nursing. (1982). *A prescriptive plan for faculty assignment, evaluation, and development*. Baltimore.

Waltz, C. F., Strickland, O. L., & Lenz, E. R. (1984). *Measurement in nursing research* (pp. 281–285). Philadelphia: F. A. Davis.

Appendix: Blockage Questionnaire

1. The school of nursing seems to recruit as many dullards as efficient people.
2. Lines of responsibility are unclear.
3. No one seems to have a clear understanding of what causes the school's problems.
4. The school is not short of skills, but they seem to be of the wrong kind.
5. It would help if people showed more interest in their jobs.
6. Good suggestions are not taken seriously.
7. Each department acts like a separate empire.
8. The administrators believe that people come to work only for money.
9. There are no clear successors to key people.
10. People do not spend adequate time planning for the future.
11. There is much disagreement about salary rates.
12. It takes too long for people to reach an acceptable standard of performance.
13. Jobs are not clearly defined.
14. There is not enough delegation.
15. Administrators do not seem to have enough time to take training seriously.
16. There are no real incentives to improve performance, so people do not bother.
17. Unconventional ideas never get a hearing.

18. Groups do not get together and work on common problems.

19. Administrators believe that tighter supervision produces increased results.

20. The school of nursing often needs to hire new administrators from the outside.

21. One of my major problems is that I do not know what is expected of me.

22. People often leave for higher salaries.

23. Employee qualifications seem to get lower each year.

24. The school of nursing reflects outdated standards and needs to be brought up to date.

25. Only top administration participates in important decisions.

26. Departments have different attitudes on training—some take it seriously, others do not.

27. Punishments seem to be handed out more frequently than rewards.

28. The school would be more successful if more risks were taken.

29. People are not prepared to say what they really think.

30. Administrators believe that people are basically lazy.

31. The school does not try to develop people for future positions.

32. Employees are told one thing and judged on another.

33. It seems that conformity brings the best reward.

34. Too many newcomers leave quickly.

35. Different parts of the school pull in different directions.

36. The school does not really know what talent is available.

37. Skills are picked up rather than learned systematically.

38. People are exploited—they are not rewarded adequately for the large amount of effort they exert.

39. Frequently, innovation is not rewarded.

40. In this school, it is every person for himself when the pressure is applied.

41. Administrators would like to revert to the days when discipline reigned supreme.

42. Administration does not identify and develop those who are potential high achievers.

43. Personal objectives have little in common with the school's aims.

44. The payment system prevents work from being organized in the best way.

45. Many employees are only barely efficient.

46. The dean has so much to do that it is impossible for her to keep in touch with everything.

47. The right information needed to make decisions is not readily available.

48. The administrators had to learn the hard way and think others should do the same.

49. People in the school do not really get a thorough explanation of how their performance is valued.

50. Competing schools seem to have brighter ideas.

51. Each administrator is responsible for his own department and does not welcome interference.

52. The only reason this school exists is to make money for the state.

53. People do not know what the school has in mind for them in the future.

54. People are judged on personal characteristics rather than on their contributions.

55. On the whole, there is no adequate method of rewarding exceptional effort.

56. There is resentment because new people seem to get the better jobs.

57. Some departments have more people than their contribution justifies.

58. The school operates on old ideas rather than on new ones.

59. Administrators are not capable of training others.

60. If the chips were down, administrators would not be fully prepared to extend themselves for the school.

61. Once something becomes an established practice, it is rarely challenged.

62. Meetings are not popular because they are generally unproductive.

63. Administration does not care whether people are happy in their work.

64. Administrative succession and development cannot be planned; there are too many variables.

65. The school's future plans are of low quality.

66. The school does not pay enough to attract sufficiently competent people.

67. There is really not much talent around.

68. All too often, important things either do not get done or get done twice.

69. Labor turnover figures are not calculated.

70. Production could be increased if the right skills were available.

71. I do not feel supported in what I am trying to do.

72. This is a dynamic age, and the school is not moving fast enough.

73. Lessons learned in one department do not get transferred to others.

74. The school does not try to make jobs interesting and meaningful.

75. Many people are trained who later join competitors.

76. Objectives are expressed in vague terms.

77. People have to work long hours to make an adequate living wage.

78. People with little or no talent and experiences are hired.

79. Some administrators are overloaded while others have it easy.

80. Employees do not know how competitive the wages are because comparative figures are not available.

81. People are not encouraged to update their skills.

82. People do not get the opportunity to contribute and, as a result, do not feel committed.

83. People do not like to "rock the boat."

84. Competition inside the school is so fierce that it becomes destructive.

85. Administrators do not think that people are interested in the quality of their working lives.

86. The experience of senior administrators is not wide enough.

87. Priorities are not clear.

88. People feel as though they work in a "second-class" school.

89. When recruiting, the school finds it difficult to sort out the wheat from the chaff.

90. There is no use talking about reorganization; attitudes are fixed.

91. Administrative-control information is not generated where it is needed.

92. Quality would be improved if the staff were more skilled.

93. The school pays below par, and people are dissatisfied.

94. Administrators are not sufficiently responsive to changes in the external environment.

95. People could help each other more, but they do not seem to care.

96. Administrators are not addressed by their first names.

97. Administrators do not believe that administrative education has much to offer them.

98. Plans seem unreal.

99. The school's total "benefits package" compares unfavorably with similar organizations.

100. The school does not have many recognized recruitment practices; individual administrators do what they think best.

101. Departments do not respect the work of other groups.

102. Administration does not recognize the cost of a dissatisfied employee.

103. It is not surprising that newcomers sometimes receive a poor impression of the school, considering the way they are treated in the first few days.

104. People would welcome more challenge in their jobs.

105. Problems are not faced openly and frankly.

106. Teams do not consciously take steps to improve the way they work together.

107. There is a lot of under-the-surface fighting between administrators.

108. Administrators are not open about the future prospects of their people.

109. Decisions are made now that should have been made months ago.

110. I, personally, feel underpaid.

DEMOGRAPHIC DATA SHEET

Please Circle the Appropriate Response

1. Employment Status
   a. Faculty
   b. Classified Staff
   c. Associate Staff
2. If Faculty
   a. Rank
      (1) Professor
      (2) Associate Professor
      (3) Assistant Professor
      (4) Instructor
      (5) Other—please specify_____
   b. Program
      (1) Undergraduate
      (2) Graduate
         (a) Career Development
         (b) CHN
         (c) Med–Surg
         (d) MCH
         (e) Primary Care
         (f) Psych
         (g) Other—please specify_____
      (3) Continuing Education
   c. Primary Responsibility
      (1) Administration
      (2) Teaching
      (3) Other—please specify_____
   d. Tenure Status
      (1) Tenured
      (2) Nontenured
3. Length of Employment with School of Nursing
   a. Less than one year
   b. 1–5 years

    c. 6–10 years
    d. 11–15 years
    e. More than 15 years

Did you complete the Blockage Questionnaire last Spring?____ Yes ____ No

4. Highest educational level attained

    a. High school diploma
    b. Associate degree
    c. Baccalaureate degree
    d. Master's degree
    e. Doctoral degree
    f. Other—please specify_____

Adapted from Woodcock, M., Francis, D. (1978). *Unblocking your organization.* San Diego, CA: University Associates, Inc. Used with permission.

3

Marketing in Nursing Organizations

Susan Bond Chambers

THE NEED FOR MARKETING IN NURSING

During the last 10 years, the environment for nursing has become increasingly complex and volatile. In educational settings, administrators are faced with declining enrollments, which are attributable to population trends resulting in a smaller pool of high school students and an increasing number of career choices available to women. Clearly, nursing is no longer a career choice for many women; other professions are open that offer higher salaries and more prestige. The problem is compounded by the fact that applicants are becoming more consumer conscious in their school choices. Students no longer view educational institutions as "ivory towers"; instead, today's nursing applicants are discriminating in their selections of nursing schools. Also, there is increased pressure for cost containment and quality of nursing education. The nursing administrator in an educational setting is forced to develop creative, entrepreneurial skills in order to cover the costs of providing nursing education. Finally, the rapidly changing health care environment has required more effort than ever for nursing education to keep "in tune" with the times.

In the clinical arena, certainly, the environment is characterized by growing attention to the supply, cost, and quality of nursing services. Administrators are faced with an imbalance in the supply and demand for nurses; they are forced to devise original techniques for attracting competent nurses to fill positions. The health care environment includes patients who are more consumer conscious in regard to delivery of health services. Nursing as the caregiver profession with the most direct patient contact is not unaware of this consciousness. Finally, the legislature is constantly monitoring and regulating the cost and quality of health services.

The increased awareness of the cost and quality of health care services has resulted in a greater number of alternatives in health care delivery and a shift to more outpatient health care services. That is, the numbers of health maintenance organizations, outpatient facilities, home health care agencies, and specialized care facilities are growing. The changing service delivery structure makes it imperative that nurses consider and attempt to control their futures in these environments while they are still being formed. More specifically, nurses need to shape the future of the nursing profession and not let it be formed by others lacking the requisite vision. Nurses need to determine which of their old roles should be maintained as well as to identify new roles that must evolve in response to the changing educational and health care scene, if the profession is to remain viable and grow.

In nursing, as in all health care professions, there is a responsibility on the part of educational and clinical administrators to provide society with an adequate supply of competent health care providers. That is, the administrators are accountable for attracting and preparing an adequate supply of competent nurses.

This chapter illustrates that marketing is a vital managerial activity in both educational and clinical nursing settings. A fully utilized strategic marketing approach provides for the ongoing monitoring of health care and health educational needs, resulting in the timely development of strategies necessary for nursing to grow in today and tomorrow's educational and clinical environment.

MARKETING DEFINED

Recently, the term *marketing* has become fashionable in nursing educational and clinical settings. While it is often seen as synonymous with promotional techniques such as selling, selling oneself, advertising, recruitment, public relations, and fund raising, these are really elements of marketing (i.e., promotion is only one component of the marketing process). Overreliance on a promotional activity, to the exclusion of other marketing components, is too limited a perspective. If organizational resources are not being utilized to the best advantage, selling or promoting the product alone will not ensure success. In educational and health service settings, managers are often guilty of considering their markets after already determining what it is they are going to do for them. The *market-driven* marketing process should not begin after the product is developed, but rather, to be effective, it must begin with an identification of needs and wants, and then lead to the development and promotion of a product that fulfills those needs and wants. In fact, if the product developed is very effective in meeting the needs of the consumer, then promotion may become a less important, even minor, activity.

Definitions of marketing that help to limit its scope include the following:

> Marketing is a total system of business activities designed to plan, price, promote and distribute want-satisfying goods and services to present and potential customers. (Stanton, 1978, p. 5)

> Marketing is the performance of business activities which direct the flow of goods and services from producer to consumer or user in order to satisfy customers and accomplish the company's objectives. . . . Marketing is concerned with designing an efficient and fair system which will direct an economy's flow of goods and services from producers to consumers and accomplish the objectives of society. (McCarthy, 1978, pp. 7–9)

> Marketing is a business strategy designed to provide information about the potentials of a service or product to consumers of a given service in order to entice the potential consumer to that given service or product. (Wise, 1981, p. 3)

These definitions narrowly define marketing as a *business activity* concerned with the flow of *goods and services* to *consumers* or *customers*. Defining marketing as a business activity excludes marketing activities performed in nonbusiness situations. For example, marketing is employed when political parties campaign for a candidate or religious groups promote causes. Another limitation with defining marketing as a business activity is the association of an activity done for the sole purpose of profits. In this light, activities undertaken in most nursing organizations would not be considered marketing, and this is certainly a fallacy.

The second limitation is that marketing is presented as concerned only with goods and services. In fact, social groups, government agencies, and religious groups often employ marketing techniques for the purpose of promoting ideas. For instance, government agencies often have employed marketing techniques when attempting to persuade communities to utilize safety belts, to not drink and drive, or to be aware of new laws.

Finally, the third limitation of these definitions is that marketing activities are directed solely to a consumer or customer. Universities perform marketing activities when attempting to raise funds via alumni; while alumni may not be considered direct customers or consumers, they certainly comprise a significant public for higher education. Similarly, hospitals or health agencies utilize marketing techniques when lobbying for a particular government action, although these marketing efforts are not directed toward consumers or customers.

The following definitions provide a broader perspective of marketing:

> Marketing encompasses exchange activities conducted by individuals and organizations for the purpose of satisfying human wants. (Enis, 1980, p. 14)

> Marketing is human activity directed at satisfying needs and wants through exchange processes. (Kotler, 1980, p. 19)

> Marketing consists of individual and organizational activities aimed at facilitating and expediting exchanges within a set of dynamic environmental forces. (Pride & Ferrell, 1980, p. 7)

Exchange

The central concept underlying each of the above definitions is that marketing is based on exchanges. Exchange is the transferring of value from one party to the other. There are four conditions that must exist in order for exchange to occur: two parties are involved, each party possesses something that is of value to the other, each party is capable of communication, and each party has the option of acceptance or rejection of the offer (Kotler, 1980, p. 20). When one is marketing nursing education, these four conditions of exchange need to exist. That is, both nursing students and representatives of the nursing school need to be involved in marketing activities. At a minimum, the nursing school offers education, while nursing students offer tuition. Communication occurs between nursing students and their school via brochures, letters, listening, reading, verbal communication, and so forth. Finally, the nursing school has the option of either accepting or rejecting students, as well as offering or not offering the educational program. Similarly, nursing students have the option of selecting or not selecting the school as well as electing or not electing to earn a nursing degree.

Nursing education institutions have numerous exchange relationships. They offer education to students in exchange for tuition, quality programs to accrediting agencies in exchange for accreditation, and employment to faculty members in exchange for their expertise. Similarly, in the clinical setting, nursing service offers nursing care to patients in exchange for the opportunity to provide for their health care needs, employment to nurses in exchange for their skills, and quality nursing care to regulatory agencies in exchange for their support. In addition, nursing education and service institutions have exchange relationships with one another: Nursing education offers nurses in-service educational opportunities, while nursing service offers nursing educators employment of students and clinical sites. The purposeful and effective management of these various exchange relations is marketing.

Wants and Needs

Also noted in the definitions is that individuals and organizations engage in exchange activities in order to satisfy their needs and wants. The terms *needs* and *wants* are often used interchangeably. A need may be defined by Webster as "a lack of something useful, required, or desired," while to want is "to feel the need of; to desire." In other words, a need is a state of condition, while a want is the awareness of the condition. As an example, students may need computer instruction; however, until they want computer instruction, its availability will not influence their decisions to attend particular schools.

Products

Needs and wants are satisfied by products. Products are divided into three categories (Enis, 1980, p. 8):

1. Goods—has tangible physical properties
2. Services—application of human skills
3. Ideas—a new concept or different way of thinking about a situation

Nursing organizations are concerned primarily with products that are services—provision of nursing care and nursing education. It is important to realize the interrelationship of product categories, since not all products can be neatly categorized. For example, the nurse practitioner must not only be concerned with marketing the service of expanded nursing care but also with the idea of a nurse performing many functions that a physician traditionally performs. The nursing education administrator must not only be concerned with marketing the service of providing education to students but also with the idea of pursuing nursing as a career.

MARKETING IN ORGANIZATIONS DEFINED

Marketing in organizations is often compartmentalized or separated from other functions. However, McKenna (1985) points out that this separation is artificial, and, in order to be successful, all functions need to consider marketing in their operations. In the nursing educational setting, this means consideration of marketing by those responsible for financial decisions, curriculum decisions, scheduling decisions, recruitment decisions, accreditation decisions, and so forth. Only when nursing educational administrators view marketing dynamically, as McKenna suggests, will the true potential of marketing on enrollment, and cost and quality of nursing education be realized.

A more specific or detailed definition of marketing as it applies to organizations is offered by Kotler and Fox (1985):

> Marketing is the analysis, planning, implementation and control of carefully formulated programs designed to bring about voluntary exchanges of values with target markets to achieve institutional objectives. Marketing involves designing the institution's offerings to meet the target markets' needs and desires, and using effective pricing, communication and distribution to inform, motivate and service the markets. (p. 7)

Key elements in this definition important for an understanding of marketing as it relates to organizations are marketing programs; target markets; target markets' needs and desires; institutional objectives; and offering design, pricing, communication, and distribution.

Marketing Programs

Marketing programs are the plans by which marketing actions are carried out to achieve the desired responses. Programs, in order to be successful, are carefully and strategically employed; they are continually analyzed, planned, implemented, and controlled. Furthermore, to ensure effectiveness, marketing activities are conducted as a series of interrelated events and not in a haphazard, fragmented manner.

Target Markets

Marketing programs are specifically designed for *target markets*. A market is a potential arena for the trading of resources (Kotler & Goldgehn, 1981), while a target market is a set of individuals or organizations who possess unique characteristics that provide for a good fit with a specific product. An organization should systematically design its product in terms of the *target markets' defined needs and desires*, not on the basis of preconceived notions regarding what the needs of the target markets are or should be. For example, if the target market for a gerontology continuing education program is nursing administrators of private urban nursing homes, the needs of this group in regard to content, learning methods, location, and scheduling need to be defined objectively in order to design the program. This dimension of the definition is in accordance with the marketing concept.

The Marketing Concept

The *marketing concept* provides the rationale for marketing simply purporting that the organization needs to be market oriented rather than product oriented. The organization should view itself as a buyer of markets, not a seller of products. In other words, the first step in marketing is identification of the needs and desires of markets rather than markets to sell an established product. Conversely, the product concept, or product-oriented approach, designs the product and then attempts to find a market to fit the product. Applying the marketing concept to education, for example, involves identifying the needs and wants of the nursing student markets, and then selecting a market and developing a product, for example—program, course, book—that fulfills these needs and achieves organizational objectives. The needs of the various publics (e.g., accrediting agencies, health care providers) as well as the students' needs are considered in this process. From an educational viewpoint, the marketing concept is akin to the *college fit theory*, which proposes that the more congruent the student's values, goals, and attitudes are with those of the college, the more likely the student will persist at that college. The college fit theory has been evaluated and supported by numerous studies (Pantages & Creedon, 1978). Hence, this theory and its evaluation provides validation of the legitimacy of the marketing concept. In nursing service, an example of the application of the marketing concept is the identification of the patient markets' needs and wants, selection of an attractive market, and the developing of the nursing care product in order to fulfill a market's needs and achieve organizational objectives. Once again, consideration is placed on all of the relevant publics in establishing the patient market's needs.

Institutional Objectives

The purpose of marketing programs is to achieve established *institutional objectives*. The institutional objectives (or mission) are the definition or rationale of the purpose and thrust of the organization. The objectives provide a framework for developing marketing programs; that is, if a nursing school's mission is to provide for the local community needs for nurses, then marketing programs should be based on achieving this mission. The marketing programs should ascertain the local needs for nurses with particular qualifications and then develop and promote programs to the community. If the mission of a clinic is to provide for the needs of the minority population, then marketing programs should be undertaken to examine the needs of this population, followed by program development and promotion.

Finally, Kotler's definition states that a set of tools—the marketing mix—*offering design (or product/design), pricing, communication and distribution* are employed to inform, motivate, and service markets. These elements of marketing are employed to develop marketing strategies designed for the target market. The marketing mix is more popularly termed the *Four Ps* of marketing—product, price, promotion, and place.

The Four Ps of Marketing

A *product* is something that is capable of satisfying a need or want (Kotler, 1980, p. 20). As stated previously, products can be classified into services, ideas or goods. As illustrated in Figure 1, nursing education and service settings may offer a variety of products. Of course, the major product of nursing educational institutions is education, and the major product of nursing service settings is nursing care. However, if a nursing school is developing a marketing program to help its graduates

Figure 1
The Four Ps of Marketing
in Nursing Education and Service

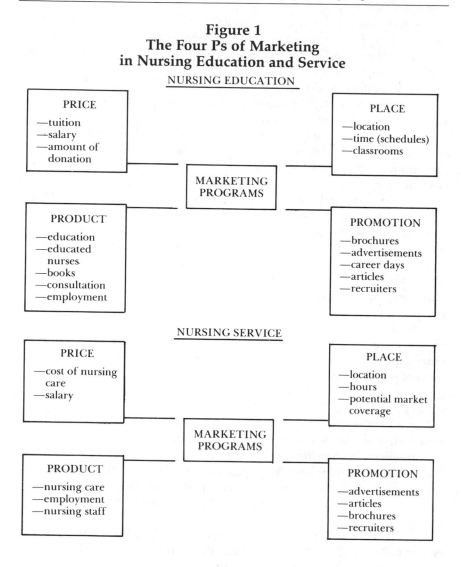

NURSING EDUCATION

PRICE
—tuition
—salary
—amount of
    donation

PLACE
—location
—time (schedules)
—classrooms

**MARKETING
PROGRAMS**

PRODUCT
—education
—educated
    nurses
—books
—consultation
—employment

PROMOTION
—brochures
—advertisements
—career days
—articles
—recruiters

NURSING SERVICE

PRICE
—cost of nursing
    care
—salary

PLACE
—location
—hours
—potential market
    coverage

**MARKETING
PROGRAMS**

PRODUCT
—nursing care
—employment
—nursing staff

PROMOTION
—advertisements
—articles
—brochures
—recruiters

find jobs, then the product being marketed is the school's graduate nurse. Similarly, if a clinic is developing a marketing program in order to attract competent nurses, then the product being marketed is nursing employment.

The group of all products offered by an organization typically is called a *product mix*. For example, a large university offers many educational programs, which are its product mix. The product mix of a hospital is all of the various health care services offered. A *product line* is a group of closely related products within a product mix. The health sciences campus is a product line of the university. The critical care unit of the hospital is one-product line. A *product item* is a distinct unit within a product line. The nursing college is a product item of the university. Coronary care is a product item of the hospital.

Price is the valuation of the product and is most often viewed in monetary terms, for example, tuition, cost of health care, price of books, and amount of donations. However, the actual charge is not the only cost (Kotler, 1982). In addition to the actual charge, there are *effort costs, psychic costs*, and *opportunity costs* (Rothman, Teresa, Kay, & Morningstar, 1983). Effort costs are the costs of the energy expended to consume the product—as an example, the time, cost, and trouble for students to commute to a nursing school. Psychic costs are the emotional costs of consuming a product—such a cost in nursing education may be the anxiety and stress a student experiences as a result of the educational experience. Opportunity costs are the costs of the benefit foregone as a result of consuming the product. The student electing to go to school full-time has bypassed the opportunity of working full-time. In some instances in nursing organizations, there are only nonmonetary aspects of products; one case would be the nursing service agency marketing to elicit volunteers—since there is no salary involved, the price viewed by the volunteer is the commitment of the effort required to do the volunteer work.

Consider the costs that make up the price of a nursing administration course to the nursing student. At a minimum, the student incurs the monetary cost of tuition and books; the effort cost of traveling to the course and the scheduling required to take the course; the opportunity cost of foregone salary and opportunity to take a different course; and the psychic cost of the stress of taking exams, completing assignments, and learning the material.

Promotion is activity undertaken in order to inform, persuade, or remind (McCarthy, 1978, p. 514). Promotional tools fall into four groups: (Kotler, 1982, pp. 354–355):

1. Advertising—any paid form of nonpersonal presentation and promotion of ideas, goods or services by an identified sponsor.

2. Sales promotion—short-term incentives to encourage purchase or sales of a product.

3. Personal selling—oral presentation in a conversation with one or

more prospective purchasers for the purpose of making sales or building goodwill.

4. Publicity—nonpersonal stimulation of demand for a product or business unit by planting commercially significant news about it in a published medium or obtaining favorable presentation of it on radio, television, or stage that is not paid for by the sponsor.

Promotional techniques are not new to nursing educational settings. For years, nursing schools have advertised programs and faculty positions, sent faculty members to high schools to recruit students, and developed brochures for programs. In nursing service settings, while promotion is a relatively new concept, its value has been recognized. This greater acceptance is validated by the increasing frequency of promotional techniques employed in service settings. In employing promotional techniques in either nursing educational or service settings, care needs to be taken to ensure that they are seen as ethical and appropriate.

Place involves considerations related to accessibility, availability, and convenience of the product. In nursing educational settings, factors such as location of the school, scheduling (time and specific locations) of courses, and number of courses offered are place considerations. In nursing service settings, factors such as location of the facility and hours of service of the facility are place considerations.

In nursing, as in many professions when applying marketing, too often the most attention is placed on only one of these tools (e.g., promotion). However, in order to be effective, it is necessary to consider all of these tools in developing marketing programs. More specifically, the nurse administrator in a clinical setting must consider the cost of nursing care, the quality of and/or manner in which nursing care is delivered, the accessibility and location of the care, and how the quality and availability of nursing care is being communicated. In nursing education settings, consideration needs to be given to the quality of the programs, the cost of the education, the locale of the school, and the manner in which the availability and quality of the nursing programs are being communicated.

MARKETING REVOLUTION

The acceptance and application of marketing principles and practices in nursing educational and clinical settings has grown dramatically, as evidenced by the proliferation of meetings, workshops, and conferences focused on marketing for nurses. In addition, the nursing literature provides validation that marketing has become more of an acceptable activity in both settings. The irony of this new "marketing revolution" in nursing is that although it is not labeled as such, to an extent marketing practices have been utilized in nursing for a number of years, albeit in a fragmented manner.

Nurses have been "data collectors." For example, numerous major studies of national scope have focused on various aspects of nursing and its future. More specifically, studies have examined the demand for and supply of nurses, the characteristics and needs of nurses, the need for nurses with particular qualifications, factors affecting the market for nurses, and future directions for the nursing profession (National League for Nursing, 1982; Balint, Menninger, & Hurt, 1983; Department of Health and Human Services, 1982, 1983; Gulack, 1983; Institute of Medicine, 1983; Lewis, 1984). These studies border on marketing research, but the additional step not undertaken in such efforts is to examine and synthesize the overall results of these studies in order to devise and implement improved marketing strategies.

In both clinical and educational settings, evaluation has been identified as an important organizational function. In the latter setting, evaluation traditionally has included, at the minimum, consideration of courses, students, alumni, faculty, programs, and curriculum. The purpose, design, and methodology of evaluation activities are similar to those of marketing research, and the utilization of the evaluation results for designing and implementing an improvement in education is similar to effecting a marketing strategy. More specifically, when a course is evaluated by students, in essence a facet of the product provided by the school is being critiqued by one of the consumers or markets of the product. This is no different in theory than when a computer company surveys its users about satisfaction with its keyboards. Furthermore, if the course evaluation findings result in restructuring the course to improve quality, it is analogous to modification of the computer keyboard to enhance quality of the product. In a clinical setting, it is not unusual for patients to be requested, on discharge, to complete a questionnaire designed to assess their satisfaction with the hospital nursing care. This is similar to when a computer company surveys its customers about satisfaction with their computer purchases.

Needs assessment is a facet of evaluation that is utilized frequently in both clinical and educational settings; it is comparable to a marketing feasibility study. For example, in the clinical arena, a needs assessment may be conducted to determine if there is a demand for a hypertensive outpatient clinic. The following would be examined: the characteristics of the population of the surrounding community and those of the hypertensive population, the extent to which the needs for such care are being met, and in what ways a clinic could better meet the needs of the hypertensive population. Similarly, a marketing feasibility study undertakes to determine the following: if a new product or service is in demand by a population, the characteristics of the population desirous of the product, how the need for this product is currently being met, and in what ways a new product would better meet the needs of the population.

In an educational setting, a needs assessment is often conducted to determine the plausibility of planning and implementing a continuing education program. One end goal of conducting such a needs assessment, and one familiar requirement in applying for continuing education units (CEUs), is to identify a target population for the program. Similarly, the marketing literature advocates the need to identify target markets for a product.

Traditionally, in educational settings, students are recruited via methods such as brochures, newspaper advertisements, career days, and faculty visits to high schools. These are all activities that can be characterized as promotion, which is one element of marketing. In addition, there have been campaigns conducted by national nursing organizations in order to portray a better "image" of nursing; this comes under the realm of promotion.

All of these activities—nursing research studies, evaluation, needs assessment, advertisement, public relations—are marketing related; however, they have not been labeled as such. More important, in nursing these activities have most often been conducted in a fragmented manner as isolated undertakings and not as interrelated events that are components of a comprehensive strategic marketing effort.

PROFIT VERSUS NONPROFIT MARKETING

The practice of marketing in nursing clinical and education settings is part of nonprofit marketing. The notion of applying marketing practices in nonprofit organizations is a relatively new one.

The unique characteristics of nonprofit organizations are what underscore the differences between marketing in a nonprofit versus profit organization. These characteristics are also the unique considerations when marketing is applied in nursing organizations. These characteristics include (Lovelock & Weinberg, 1978, pp. 416–420):

1. Multiple publics.
2. Multiple objectives.
3. Services rather than physical goods.
4. Public scrutiny.

Table 1 contrasts these characteristics for a profit versus nonprofit organization.

Nonprofit organizations have multiple publics to consider. A *public* may be defined as a distinct group of people and/or organizations that have an actual or potential impact on the organization (Kotler & Goldgehn, 1981). A public is determined a market when it is thought of in terms of trading something of value (Kotler & Goldgehn, 1981).

Nonprofit organizations have at the least two major publics—clients and funders. Hence, nonprofit organizations need to be concerned with both resource attraction and allocation. In nursing education settings, there are multiple publics. At a minimum, the publics include potential students, current students, alumni, the nursing profession, parents, faculty, donors, accrediting agencies, the community, nursing organizations, health care provider agencies, other nursing education providers, and legislators. For example, the publics for a nursing department of a hospital illustrates that nursing clinical settings publics include, but are not limited to, clients, the community, local government, reimbursement organizations, professional associations, trustees, donors, suppliers, other health care professionals, volunteers, patients' families, the nursing profession, legislators, and other health care provider organizations. While it could be argued that business organizations also have multiple publics to consider, their focus is normally to market to one public—the customer. In nursing educational and clinical settings, all of the various publics need to be considered when developing marketing programs. The importance of a particular public depends upon the individual situation. For example, it can be surmised that in a publicly funded nursing school, the importance of the local community would be more so than in a privately funded nursing school. Attempting to fulfill the needs of the various publics makes the practice of marketing in nursing organizations more complex than in profit-motivated organizations.

The second factor distinguishing nonprofit organizations is that it is necessary to pursue several objectives simultaneously. In nursing edu-

Table 1
Considerations in Marketing for a Profit versus Nonprofit Organization

Characteristics	Nonprofit	Profit
Number of publics	Multiple—at the minimum clients and funders	Primarily one—customer or consumers
Number of objectives	Multiple—number and importance of each depends on situation	Primarily one—to obtain a profit
Type of products	Usually services or ideas—are intangible, inseparable, variable, and perishable	Usually goods—more controllable than services and ideas
Level of public scrutiny	High—because providers of public services	Low—because are rarely providers of public services

cational settings, the objectives may consist of the following: recruiting sufficient numbers of quality students, meeting the needs of health care providers for nurses, meeting the needs of the local community for nurses, enhancing the reputation of the school, fulfilling accreditation requirements, and so forth. In clinical settings, the nursing objectives may be to increase collaboration with other health care professionals, decrease cost of nursing services, decrease turnover rate of nursing staff, improve patient satisfaction, increase awareness of nursing services, and so forth. Whatever the objectives established for a nonprofit organization are, devising marketing strategies is more difficult than when the objective is merely profit motivated. Often, it becomes necessary to decide on the relative importance of the objectives in establishing a marketing program.

Most nonprofit organizations provide services rather than physical goods. Services have the characteristics of being intangible, inseparable, variable, and perishable. Nursing schools offer an intangible service—education; the nursing faculty member is inseparable from the course taught; the quality of the education is variable in that faculty members vary in quality, and the education is perishable in that if enrollment drops, you cannot save the educational resources for the next year's students. In the clinical arena, nurses offer the intangible service of nursing care, the nurse is inseparable from the care provided, the care is variable in that the nurses vary in competence and expertise, and the nursing care is perishable in that if there are unfilled beds in the hospital, the nursing care cannot be stored from day to day. These characteristics make marketing a more difficult task.

Finally, nonprofit organizations are usually prone to more public scrutiny since they usually provide public services. Whether or not the institution is public or private, the provision of nursing education and nursing care are considered within the realm of public services. The activities of nursing, clinical, and educational institutions are under close public scrutiny; hence, the marketing activities of these institutions are also under close public scrutiny.

Thus far, marketing has been defined, its various components have been presented, and its applicability to nursing settings has been illustrated. However, the manner in which a marketing approach is implemented within an organization has not been provided. An approach for implementing the marketing function within an organization is the strategic marketing process.

INTERRELATIONSHIP OF STRATEGIC MARKETING AND STRATEGIC PLANNING

Strategic implies progressive thinking to optimize future operations in light of the organization's service characteristics and trends (Hillestad & Berry, 1980). The strategic marketing process is, in essence, the framework for the conduct of strategic marketing activities within an organization. In other words, strategic marketing is the progressive planning and management of marketing activities in order to maximize organizational strengths and achieve organizational objectives.

Strategic marketing and planning are often presented as synonymous terms. In fact, it is not unusual for strategic planning to be identified as strategic market planning and/or for the two approaches to be presented as one process or approach. It is certainly not inappropriate for strategic marketing and planning to be presented as one comprehensive, cohesive process, given their reciprocal nature. This book presents strategic planning and strategic marketing as separate, yet parallel, activities in order to provide the reader with an in-depth discussion of each process.

The interrelationship of strategic marketing and planning is two-dimensional. On one dimension, strategic planning is market based (i.e., relies on marketing inputs or information). On another dimension, strategic planning provides direction for the marketing function. More specifically, the objectives and goals that result from the strategic-planning process provide the strategic-marketing effort direction for marketing activities. Hence, the two processes are essentially interdependent. Strategic planning is dependent upon marketing to provide necessary information upon which to base planning decisions, and strategic marketing relies on strategic planning to provide guidance and/or boundaries for the conduct of marketing activities.

It has been recognized that the failure of marketing efforts can often be tied to the lack of an effective strategic-planning process. LaTour (1984, p. 5) purports, "Most organizations have failed to develop an effective corporate strategic planning process which could provide appropriate direction for the marketing function. . . . The basic role of marketing management is to assure that the organization's strategic objectives are satisfied through a customer-oriented approach to service provisions." An important point has also been made that if marketing is tied to strategic-planning goals and objectives of the organization, there will be less criticism because marketing activities are not conducted for growth for growth's sake or aggrandizement (Gallattscheck, 1981).

Stated more specifically, strategic marketing's contribution to the strategic-planning process is the generation, analysis, and provision of information related to market trends and demands, environmental influences, competitor strengths and weaknesses, and internal strengths and weaknesses. This information is used to aid in the defining of long-term strategic objectives for the organization within which the marketing function operates. As will become apparent in the following sections, this information is used to make strategic-marketing decisions as well. One particularly valuable marketing input into the strategic-planning process is portfolio analysis.

PORTFOLIO ANALYSIS—A MARKETING INPUT TO STRATEGIC PLANNING

Portfolio analysis is a method to examine the market positions of an organization's offerings. Its purpose is to determine the extent to which existing products are likely to support organizational objectives and to assure that the portfolio is balanced, so that all objectives are met (LaTour, 1984).

To conduct a portfolio analysis, strategic business units (SBUs) are identified and analyzed on a quantitative continuum that is meaningful to the organization. Strategic business units are entities within an organization that are unique and separable to some extent from each other. The entities or units are usually separable on the basis of markets served or products offered. Examples of SBUs in nursing education are individual nursing programs (e.g., baccalaureate, masters, doctoral, continuing education) of a nursing school and/or concentrations within an individual nursing program (e.g., administration, clinical specialization). In a nursing service environment, SBUs may be departments within the hospital (e.g., obstetrics, coronary care, pediatrics, emergency) or geographical areas served by the home health agency.

There are several prototypes for portfolio analysis. The model most appropriate for nursing organizations is the General Electric (GE) Portfolio Grid, illustrated in Figure 2. The vertical axis represents market attractiveness, and the horizontal axis represents organizational strength. Each axis is a composite index of a variety of factors. Suggested factors by GE for market attractiveness include the following: market size, market growth rate, profit margin, competitive intensity,

Figure 2
General Electric Portfolio Approach

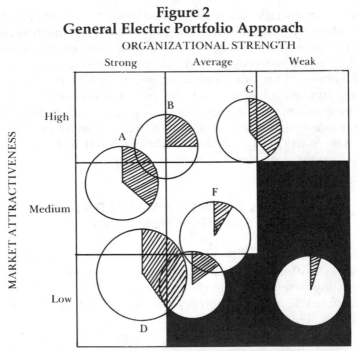

[1]Used with permission from Kotler, P. (1982). *Marketing for nonprofit organizations.* (2nd. ed.). Englewood Cliffs, NJ: Prentice-Hall.

cyclicality (the extent to which demand is stable), seasonality (the extent to which demand is seasonal), scale economics (the extent to which unit costs decrease with volume), and learning curve (the extent to which costs decrease as experience with the SBU increases). The model suggests the following factors to be included in the organizational index: program quality, efficiency level, market knowledge, and marketing effectiveness (Kotler, 1982).

In order to operationalize the model, each factor within the composite index is ranked according to importance to the organization. The SBUs are then rated on each factor and are plotted on to the grid. The size of the circle is proportionate to the size of the industry of the SBU, and the size of the pie slice represents the SBU's market share. General Electric defines three zones on the grid of green, yellow and red. The green zone represents the upper-left portion of the grid, where SBUs are in attractive markets and where there is organizational strength. The yellow zone is the diagonal of the grid, where SBUs are at a middle level of attractiveness. The red zone is the lower-right area, where SBUs are low in attractiveness.

In order to conceptualize the usefulness of the GE portfolio model, it is useful to examine the application by Zallocco, Joseph, and Dremus (1984) of the GE model to a hospital setting. Figure 3 illustrates their application. They defined market attractiveness as being composed of five major criteria:

Rank	Market Attractiveness Criteria
1	*Market characteristics*—size, growth rate, relationship to existing or other planned programs and sensitivity to price, service, features, etc.
2	*Financial factors*—profit margin, economics of scale and experience, inputs and trends in government financial participation, inputs and trends in third party financial participation.
3	*Competitive intensity.*
4	*Technology*—maturity, complexity.
5	*Socioenvironmental factors.*

Zallocco et al. defined organizational (hospital) strength as being composed of six major criteria:

Rank	Organizational Strength Criteria
1	*Centrality to mission.*
2	*Program quality.*
3	*Financial factors*—capacity utilization, profit margins achieved, fixed/variable costs.
4	*Marketing effectiveness*—relative market share, marketing influence, competitive position.
5	*Organizational skills*—management skills, responsiveness and flexibility, relationships with environmental organizations.
6	*Differentiation*—reputation, technology.

A 10-point scale (10 = high, 1 = low) was used to rate each identified SBU on the criteria. The scores were inverted so that the directions of the ratings were consistent with the ranked weights (the lower the score, the more favorable the rating). The ratings and the rank of the factor are multiplied, and then all factors are summed in order to get a composite score on market attractiveness and on hospital strength. Zallocco et al. defined the size of the circle as proportional to revenue generated.

Kotler (1982) suggests strategies for each zone, that is, the green or favorable zone SBUs should be targeted for investment and growth, the yellow or moderate zone SBUs should be maintained, and SBUs in the red zone should be terminated or harvested (divested). Of course, these are general guidelines, and the actual decisions depend on individual situations.

The advantage of employing the GE model over others is the ability to design the model to fit individual organizations. The GE portfolio analysis not only assists the administrator in making strategic decisions in regard to SBUs, but it can also be used to plot competitors' SBUs. In this way, the model can be used to choose competitive positions.

THE STRATEGIC MARKETING PROCESS

The approach to strategic marketing for nursing education and service advocated in this book is a modification of the strategic-marketing process proposed by Kotler (1980). The differences between the two approaches are explicated in Table 2. The modifications were made to Kotler's approach in order to:

Figure 3
Portfolio Grid for Hospitals

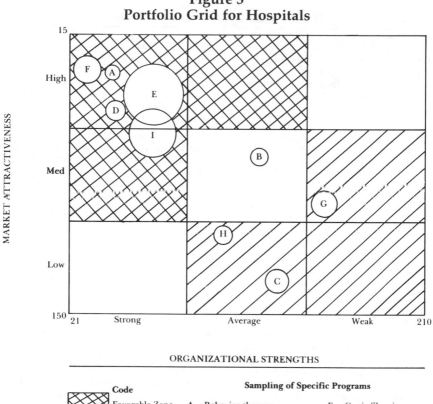

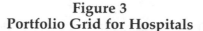

From Zallocco, R. L., Joseph, W. B., Doremus, H. (1984). Strategic market planning for hospitals. *Journal of Health Care Marketing, 4*(2), 19–28. Published by American Marketing Association.

1. Design a strategic marketing process appropriate for an organization as a whole (i.e., Kotler focuses on development of one product or SBU within an organization).

2. Emphasize and further explicate the role of the marketing analysis step in the strategic-marketing process.

3. Design a strategic-marketing process more useful for a first-time integration of the marketing function within an organization.

Table 2
The Strategic Marketing Process

Kotler (1980, pp. 80–90)	Modified
Market Opportunity Analysis—develop an attractive set of opportunities for the organization in which the organization is likely to enjoy a differential advantage	Marketing Systems Development—delegation of responsibility, explication of objectives, allocation of resources, formulation of time frames, establishment of information system for the marketing effort
Target Market Selection—market segmentation; selection of the most attractive market to serve	Marketing Analysis—identification of information needs and the collection of secondary and primary data that addresses the information need; the analysis is organized into three phases: organizational, competitive, and market
Competitive Positioning—development of a general idea of what kind of offer to make to the target market in relation to competitors' offers	Marketing Opportunity and Threat Analysis—determination of the major opportunities and threats that exist
Marketing Systems Development—development of a marketing organization, information system, and control system that promises to accomplish the organization's objectives in the target market	Target Market Selection—market segmentation; selection of the most attractive markets to serve
Marketing Plan Development—development of a marketing plan for the target market; elements include: (1) situation analysis (summary of recent performance, presentation of trends and issues), (2) marketing objectives and goals, (3) marketing strategies, action program, and budget	Marketing Plan Development—development of a marketing plan for the organization and individual SBUs; elements include: (1) a statement of market position, (2) marketing objectives and goals, and (3) marketing strategies action programs and budget
Plan Implementation and Control—assignment of goals and tasks to specific persons to be accomplished within specific time; control for achievement of marketing and organization's objectives, efficiency, and profitability	Plan Implementation and Control—assignment of responsibilities for accomplishment in order to achieve the objectives of the marketing plan; evaluation of the marketing plan's effectiveness and efficiency

More specifically, Kotler's approach involves six steps:

1. *Market Opportunity Analysis*—development of a set of opportunities for the organization.
2. *Target Market Selection*—examination of the markets for each opportunity and selection of the most attractive market to serve.

3. *Competitive Positioning*—development of a general idea of what kind of offer to make to the target market in relation to competitor's offers.

4. *Marketing Systems Development*—development of a marketing organization and systems to accomplish the objectives in the target market.

5. *Marketing Plan Development*—formulation of a plan that spells out goals, strategies, and tactics to gain the results the organization is seeking in the target market.

6. *Plan Implementation and Control*—assignment of goals and tasks to be accomplished and control for achievement of marketing and organizational objectives.

The modified model focuses on all of the organization's existing and potential products. This is due to the perspective that, in many instances in nursing education and service, it is more effective and efficient to consider all of these products simultaneously. Increased efficiency is best illustrated by considering marketing analysis activities. For example, it is very likely that it would be more efficient to collect data concerning educational facilities from students of all nursing programs instead of focusing on one program. Similarly, in the hospital setting, it would be more efficient to collect patient demographic information for patients of all departments in the same manner than for each department to design and implement its own collection process. In more general terms, it is simply more economical for the nursing organization to share marketing resources. Furthermore, the perspective of the organization as a whole is important, so that the interrelationships among products are considered and that the manner in which all products contribute to the organizational image is examined. It is easier, for example, for a nursing school to develop a reputation for educational excellence if all of their education programs are working toward this goal. If one program is initiating social activities and promoting the social aspects of the program, while another program is providing forums for discussing nursing issues and promoting the program as the one serious about education, the reputation of the school as a whole will certainly be confused. The modified model, in contrast to Kotler's model, begins with Marketing Systems Development in order to establish networks for implementation of a marketing effort. The next step is Marketing Analysis, which involves information collection in regard to a variety of aspects of the organization's products. This step was added because it is important that the nursing school or nursing service agency place priority on being knowledgeable about trends and factors that influence the provision of nursing care and education. The remaining four steps of the process—Market Opportunity and Threat Analysis, Target Market Selection, Marketing Plan Development, and Plan Implementation and Control, are basically structured the same as Kotler's model; the only modification is that the focus is on the organization as a whole, instead of on one product or SBU. The Competitive Positioning step proposed by Kotler was not included in the modified model, since consideration of competitor's offerings is a facet of the Target Market Selection step of the modified model.

A more detailed illustration of the strategic-marketing process proposed by this book is provided in Figure 4. As depicted in the figure, the process involves a series of six sequential steps. The process is continuous, and each step depends upon the activities conducted in previous steps. The definitions of the steps are:

1. *Marketing Systems Development*—the establishment and maintenance of the marketing function within the organization.

2. *Marketing Analysis*—the determination of marketing information needs and the collection and analysis of data to address the information needs.

3. *Market Opportunity and Threat Analysis*—the synthesis of the information uncovered during the marketing analysis in order to determine the major opportunities and threats for the organization.

4. *Target Market Selection*—determination of the most attractive markets to serve.

5. *Marketing Plan Development*—development of a written document that outlines marketing objectives for the organization, marketing strategies, actions to be taken to achieve objectives, and a budget.

6. *Plan Implementation and Control*—assignment of responsibility and resources in order to effectively implement the marketing plan and ongoing evaluation of the marketing plan's effectiveness.

Marketing Systems Development

Step 1—Marketing Systems Development.   This procedure involves the activities necessary for establishing and maintaining the marketing function within the organization. Establishment of the marketing function within the organization involves:

Figure 4
The Strategic Marketing Process

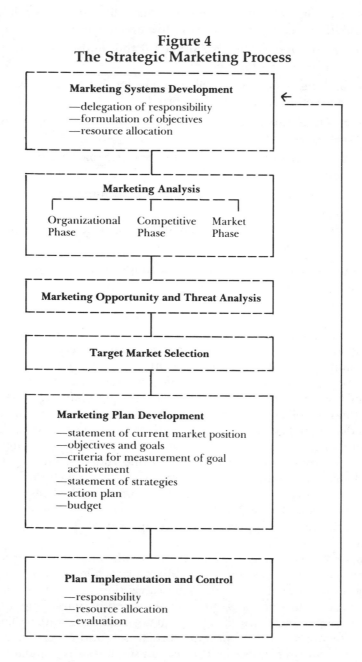

Marketing Systems Development

—delegation of responsibility
—formulation of objectives
—resource allocation

Marketing Analysis

Organizational   Competitive   Market
Phase   Phase   Phase

Marketing Opportunity and Threat Analysis

Target Market Selection

Marketing Plan Development

—statement of current market position
—objectives and goals
—criteria for measurement of goal
  achievement
—statement of strategies
—action plan
—budget

Plan Implementation and Control

—responsibility
—resource allocation
—evaluation

1. Determining at what level(s) marketing will be placed within the organization, i.e., where on the organizational chart.
2. Identifying who will be responsible for the conduct of marketing activities within the organization.
3. Establishing a system by which marketing information is obtained and marketing activities are reported.
4. Determining the objectives or defining the desired outcomes of the marketing effort.
5. Identifying the time frame in which specific marketing activities will be conducted.
6. Allocating resources to support accomplishment of the objectives within the time period.
7. Insuring that a marketing orientation is provided to personnel at all levels of the organization.

In nursing education and service settings, as in most organizations, the marketing function is usually most appropriately placed at the top-management level of the organizational chart. At the minimum, top-level-administrative support and involvement is important because deans, vice presidents of nursing, CEOs, and so forth, possess the authority and perspective of the total organization necessary to successfully implement the marketing effort. Furthermore, since strategic marketing provides inputs to strategic planning, it is important that the administrators who are involved with strategic planning work closely with those involved with strategic marketing. It should be noted, however, that the marketing function needs to be supportive of all levels of the organization. In this manner, marketing should be thought of as more of a supportive function than a line function on the organizational chart. Marketing needs to be consistently applied throughout all levels of the organization. For example, the individual responsible for marketing should be supportive of a faculty member developing a new course, as well as supportive of development of a new doctoral program.

Nursing educational institutions often subsume marketing activities under the role of the admissions director. While there is certainly a connection between the two functions, caution needs to be exercised, since these individuals are often not prepared in marketing or because of past experiences are likely to equate marketing with selling techniques (e.g., recruitment, program brochures, and advertisements).

In both nursing service and education settings, it is popular to set up a marketing committee. While committees can be advantageous in that a variety of perspectives are available, committees often run into problems when trying to establish a consensus, and, subsequently, productivity can be hampered. A committee can be useful, however, in identifying marketing information sources as well as in brainstorming marketing strategies.

Probably the most effective method for integrating marketing within the nursing organization is to designate one individual as having ultimate responsibility for marketing activities who reports to a top administrator, and to establish a marketing committee that supports this individual. This method would allow for the advantages of top-administrative support, the advantages of a committee's input, and the advantages of having one individual with ultimate responsibility for marketing. However, the marketing function is integrated into the organization, it is important that the job responsibilities for individuals involved are clearly defined in order to avoid duplication of effort and/or vital activities not being accomplished. One technique for accomplishing this goal is responsibility charting, which is described in detail in chapter 6.

The manner in which the marketing function relates to other departments is also established during the Marketing Systems Development step. In order to be effective, it is important that there is a reciprocal relationship between marketing and other departments of the organization. In nursing education settings, the individual with responsibility for marketing will need to work closely with admissions, finance, development, and public relations offices, and he or she will rely on these departments' cooperation. In nursing clinical settings, the marketing function is aligned closely with finance, records, public relations, and admissions offices. It is useful to document formally (i.e., in writing) the manner in which these departments are to interact and how and what information will be shared. In fact, one perspective is that it is crucial that the individual with responsibility for marketing should have the responsibility for coordinating all of the marketing functions (including, but not limited to, admissions and public relations) (Kotler & Goldgehn, 1981). While it may appear simplistic that these functions need to relate to one another, the importance becomes clearer when it is considered that in education, for example, it is not uncommon for the heads of the admissions, finance, development, and public relations departments to report to different people (Barton & Treadwell, 1978).

Prior to implementing any marketing activities, objectives for the strategic marketing effort should be defined. The objectives, once identified and agreed upon by those involved, establish the scope and expected outcomes of the marketing effort. The objectives should be attainable and realistic; for example, a nursing school may define the following as one objective for the marketing effort: Within one year of the start-up date of the marketing effort, a marketing plan will have been developed and approved by the dean.

In a clinical agency, the following may be an objective for the strategic-marketing effort: Based on results of an objective-marketing analysis, a competitive position statement for the home health department will be identified.

A time frame for accomplishing each objective needs to be devised and disseminated. As with any activity, this device aids in keeping the marketing effort timely and also communicates to those involved the expectations for the effort. A valuable technique is Gantt Charting, which is described in chapter 6.

Resources should be allocated for the marketing effort to support the accomplishment of the objectives within the time frame. Resources necessary may include secretarial assistance, consultant fees, computer support, research analyst time, space, supplies, and so forth. It is crucial that when identifying the objectives, time frames, and necessary resources for the marketing function, the administrator try to be sure the expectations are realistic so that the marketing activities do not become ends in themselves.

Finally, and probably most important, the understanding of and support for marketing activities needs to be acquired by individuals at all levels of the organization. The *understanding* of marketing precedes implementation, and, in fact, it is more important to understand the marketing process and relationships than to be concerned with its organizational structure (Miaoulis et al., 1985). The marketing concept not only needs to be understood by members of the organization but also needs to be accepted and supported. In simple terms, the marketing effort needs to be marketed. The need to develop an understanding and support of marketing is especially prevalent in nursing organizations, for several reasons:

1. The majority of personnel are likely to equate marketing with selling and, hence, more often than not, view marketing as an unethical activity.
2. Since marketing activities may be initiated for the first time, and, since marketing may be viewed as a change agent, the organization needs to be prepared to expect change (Gollattscheck, 1981).

3. The success of the marketing effort relies on the cooperation of a variety of personnel in collecting marketing data, devising marketing strategies, and implementing the marketing plan; if these personnel have an understanding and belief in marketing, their cooperation will most likely be more productive.

Marketing Analysis

Step 2—Marketing Analysis. This is the most crucial step of the process, since its purpose is to provide objective information to be used in making marketing decisions and developing marketing programs. Conducting a marketing analysis involves identifying marketing information needs and collecting secondary data (existing information) and primary data (development of new information) that address the information needs. A marketing-information need is simply a question that, if addressed, provides useful information for making marketing decisions.

This step begins with establishing the marketing-information system or what information is necessary to enable the organization to make objective marketing decisions and develop marketing programs. The marketing analysis and, subsequently, the marketing-information system are organized into three phases: organizational, market, and competitive.

The organizational phase involves auditing the organization's resources in order to evaluate the strengths and weaknesses of the organization. The collective information needs or questions are designed to answer the questions, "What does the organization do best?" and "What does the organization need to improve upon?"

The market phase involves the assessment of the current and potential markets for the organization's products. The focus is on identifying the needs and characteristics of markets, the needs of influential publics, the future trends for products, and environmental and societal influences.

During the competitive phase, others who offer similar products are identified. The collective information needs are designed to answer the questions, "What are the competitors offering?" "In what areas does the organization perform better than the competitor?" and "In what areas does the competitor perform better than the organization?"

In the design of the marketing-information system, all information needs that potentially influence marketing decisions should be included; however, it should be understood that all of the marketing questions or information needs cannot possibly be addressed at once. If unrealistic expectations are made, the marketing analysis will become inexpedient and untimely. Those information needs that are most critical are focused on initially.

In most nursing organizations, there are several levels of analysis. The levels of analysis define the boundaries of the marketing analysis and are best illustrated by a Marketing Analysis Grid. Figure 5 is a marketing analysis grid for a nursing school. Two different levels of analysis are depicted; one is an educational program, which includes levels of all of the educational programs, the baccalaureate program, the baccalaureate-generic program, the baccalaureate-RN program, and so forth. The other level of analysis is geographic and for this particular school includes local, regional, and national geographic levels. The usefulness of the Marketing Analysis Grid is that it clarifies the scope and type of information to be collected. That is, in this particular example, information would be collected that speaks to:

- Organizational information needs for the baccalaureate program on a local level.
- Organizational information needs for the baccalaureate program on a regional level.
- Organizational information needs for the baccalaureate program on a national level.
- Market information needs for the baccalaureate program on a local level.
- Market information needs for the baccalaureate program on a regional level, etc.

While most profit-motivated organizations have to rely on primary data collection, nursing organizations have the advantage of having access to a variety of secondary data sources. In health care, and nursing specifically, there are numerous studies conducted by researchers; private organizations; and local, state, and federal government agencies that address marketing questions. The nursing literature also provides information on marketing issues. Internally, nursing educational organizations collect evaluation data, conduct needs assessments, keep admissions records, prepare accreditation reports, keep minutes from meetings, and so forth. In clinical settings, nurses conduct quality assurance activities, evaluate services and personnel, take minutes from meetings, keep patient records, prepare accreditation reports, and so forth. These already-established internal mechanisms are useful collec-

Figure 5
Marketing Analysis Grid

Phases of the Marketing Analysis

Levels of Analysis: Programs

	All Nursing Programs	BSN	BSN/RN	BSN/Generic	MSN	PhD	CE	Levels of Analysis: Geographic
1. Information Needs for the Organizational Phase								Locally
								Regionally
								Nationally
2. Information Needs for the Market Phase								Locally
								Regionally
								Nationally
3. Information Needs for the Competitive Phase								Locally
								Regionally
								Nationally

tively for the marketing analysis. All of these secondary information sources are exhausted before designing and implementing primary data collection methods in order to keep the analysis cost-effective and timely.

After secondary data is exhausted, information needs not addressed adequately are identified and prioritized. That is, information needs that are deemed essential to development of marketing strategies are ranked in order of importance. Primary data collection methods can then be designed to address these information needs.

Specific examples, techniques, and methods for designing and implementing the marketing information system, secondary data collection, and primary data collection are provided in chapter 4.

Marketing Opportunity and Threat Analysis

Step 3—Marketing Opportunity and Threat Analysis. This procedure entails the synthesis and interpretation of information collected during the marketing analysis. The goal of the marketing opportunity and threat analysis is to determine, based on marketing data, what major opportunities and threats exist for the organization in providing its various products. An opportunity for the organization is consistent with its objectives. A threat is an occurrence or trend that has potential adverse effects on the organization's ability to fulfill its objectives.

Criteria for determining whether or not opportunities and threats are major include:

1. The extent to which the organization is capable of fulfilling or taking advantage of the opportunity or altering the threat.
2. The extent to which the opportunity or threat is occurring or will occur.

These criteria are designed to focus the analysis on only those opportunities and threats that the organization is most capable of acting upon. For instance, if there is opportunity for a continuing education offering in utilization of microcomputers in the hospital setting, but the nursing school does not have faculty with expertise in this area or the computer facilities necessary (and neither resource is readily accessible), the opportunity is not a major one. If a community health center has a neighboring nursing home, the opportunity exists to fulfill the nursing home patients' health maintenance needs. However, if none of the nurses in the community health center are prepared in gerontology, then this is not a major opportunity.

Once identified, the major opportunities and threats for the organization should be prioritized utilizing the criteria described above. This allows the organization to decide upon marketing positions in an objective manner, that is, the strongest opportunities are focused on in development of the marketing plan, and strategies are developed to alter the strongest threats.

Target Market Selection

Step 4—Target Market Selection. This procedure is the identification of the most attractive markets to serve. The opportunity and threat analysis sets the framework for target market selection. More specifically, the major opportunities and threats identified are used in concert with information regarding current and potential markets of the organization in order to select target markets.

To make this selection, the market is segmented. In order to accomplish the segmentation, the total market for a product is subdivided, based on differences in requirements, demographics, or other critical characteristics (Kotler, 1980). Market segmentation allows for analyzing the needs of different markets for products based on their unique characteristics.

The concept of market segmentation is based upon the propositions that (1) consumers are different, (2) differences in consumers are related to differences in market behavior, and (3) segments of consumers can be isolated within the overall market (Lovelock, 1977). As an illustration of market segmentation, the total market for a baccalaureate program for the returning registered nurse may be subdivided into the following segments:

1. 20–30 years old, married, suburban dwellers, desire part-time day and independent study, work full-time.

2. 30–40 years old, married with children, suburban dwellers, desire full-time day study, work part-time, have approximately 10 years of nursing experience.

3. 20–30 years old, single, urban dwellers, desire part-time night study, work full-time, desire social activities.

These markets may be further subdivided into those who are:

1. hard workers and high achievers (strive for and earn a 4.0 grade-point average).

2. interested in just getting by (satisfied with a 3.0).

3. hard workers and low achievers (strive for a 4.0 but earn a 3.0).

This example illustrates only a limited number of potential segments. The subdivisions can be numerous, depending on the knowledge of the markets and the degree that the markets are heterogeneous. There is no right way to segment a market (Kotler, 1982). Several variables may need to be considered before one identifies the most meaningful market segmentation. Variables should be considered to the extent they affect the manner in which a product is consumed. For education, as an example, employment status may be a far more salient segmentation than sex because of its greater impact on the delivery of an educational program. The degree to which the segment clearly exists should also be considered. Once the markets are segmented, the organization selects those markets that are most attractive. The criteria for selection include:

1. The organization's ability to fulfill the needs of that segment.
2. The degree to which the organization is better able to attract the segment than its competitors.
3. The potential size of the segment.
4. The ability to reach the segment.

As can be seen from the second criterion, the organization needs to consider its competitive position strategy when selecting target markets. Competitive positioning is the art of developing and communicating meaningful differences between one organization's offer and the offer of competitors serving the same target market (Kotler, 1982, p. 106). A competitive position strategy is the decision of what type of offer to make in relation to competitors' offers. In developing a competitive positioning strategy, the organization focuses on how to position its product relative to the competitors' products or how to differentiate the product from the competitors' products. The focus is not necessarily on "cut-throat" competition, but instead on providing a product that is different and meets a unique market need (more popularly termed a *market niche*). In the example, if a competitor is offering a traditional program for the registered nurses returning for their bachelor of nursing science (BSN), the school may want to offer a fast-track program that leads to the master of nursing science (MSN) and targets nurses with nonnursing degrees.

Marketing Plan Development

Step 5—Marketing Plan Development. This plan involves the establishment of marketing objectives, and subsequent development of programs in order to fulfill the objectives. These objectives and programs are explicated in a marketing plan, which is a formal, comprehensive document that includes a statement of current market position, long- and short-range marketing objectives and goals, a statement of marketing strategies, an action plan to achieve strategies, and a budget for implementation of the marketing plan.

The statement of current market position, also termed situation analysis, is an overview of the organization's current standing in the marketplace and includes the pertinent findings that resulted from the marketing analysis, and marketing opportunity and threat analysis. More specifically, the following are included in a statement of current market position: a summary of the markets served by the organization, the performance of the organization in these markets, the market opportunities and threats, the strengths and weaknesses of the organization, the strengths and weaknesses of the competitors, and the marketing opportunities and threats. The statement of current market position not only provides information on organizational performance, but it also provides a summary of information that led to development of marketing objectives and goals.

Marketing objectives and goals are stated in both the long-term (5–10 years) and short-term (1–3 years) in order to ensure that the marketing efforts are continuous and comprehensive. Objectives and goals should be written so that they are:

1. A product of the previous marketing steps—each objective and goal should be linked with a marketing opportunity or threat.

2. Attainable—objectives and goals should be realistic so that the organization can achieve them.

3. Measurable—the objectives and goals need to be in terms so that evaluation of performance in achieving objectives can be measured.

An example of a long-term marketing objective and goal for a community health center may be the following:

LT Objective—to develop a reputation for serving the community's health promotion needs.
LT Goal—within five years, the majority of the new patients of the center will have already heard of the health promotion activities and/or thrust of the center.

The short-term objectives and goals corresponding to these long-term objectives and goals might be as follows:

ST Objective—to increase the number and success of the health promotion activities of the center.

ST Goal—within two years, three new health promotion activities will have been developed and introduced.

Marketing strategies are the means by which objectives are achieved. In the marketing plan, a statement of marketing strategy may also indicate why a particular plan of action was chosen in addition to outlining how the attainment of the objective will occur. Following is an example of a marketing strategy:

> *Marketing strategy*—As revealed by the marketing analysis, there are few activities for the community that focus on health promotion, and many members of the community have expressed an interest in health promotion. In addition, it is documented that the community does not view the center as a significant contributor to the health of the community. Hence, development of programs for health promotion will serve to both fulfill an unmet community need and to heighten the reputation of the center. Since providing health promotion services will be a new role for the center, emphasis needs to be placed on creating awareness of the new services.

Action plans are composed of specific tactics or steps to be undertaken in order to achieve the marketing objectives and identify the individual responsible for each tactic.

An example of some tactics to achieve the marketing strategy objectives would be as follows:

Tactics	Individual Responsible

1. Develop a "Quit Smoking" class, i.e.:
  (a) Determine the cost of an instructor, supplies, etc.
  (b) Using information available, determine the best time to offer the class.
  (c) Based on (a), determine a price or tuition for the course.
	Assistant to the director

2. Promote the "Quit Smoking" class to the community.
  (a) Contact local newspaper for free publicity articles.
  (b) Develop a flyer describing the program.
  (c) Send flyers to local MDs (general practitioners, cardiologists, etc.), hospitals, and businesses for posting.
	Director
	Assistant to the director
	Secretary

Finally, a budget is estimated for the cost of implementing the marketing plan. Procedures and techniques for devising a budget are provided in chapter 6.

Plan Implementation and Control

Step 6—Plan Implementation and Control.   This is the final step of the strategic-marketing process. Plan implementation involves the assignment of duties and responsibilities in order to carry out the marketing plan. While one person should have responsibility for the coordination of the implementation of the marketing plan, it is necessary that tasks be delegated and that administrators and staff work as a team in a concerted effort. The potential for breakdowns and duplication of effort should be alleviated by developing detailed tactics and responsibility charts (see chapter 6) for implementation of each element of the plan. As described in the preceding section, the individual with responsibility for each tactic can be designated in the marketing plan document.

Control involves evaluation of the marketing plan's effectiveness, efficiency, and cost. It is important to evaluate continually strategies and action plans for their effectiveness, so that alterations can be made in a timely manner. Control mechanisms are provided for in the marketing plan by developing criteria for measurement of goal achievement. It is necessary, however, to designate an individual to be responsible and accountable for control of the marketing plan.

The strategic-marketing process is an ongoing systematic process, which, once it is implemented for the first time, requires continual updating and monitoring. The strategic-marketing process is a vital managerial activity, which if implemented to its fullest extent in nursing organizations, will aid in ensuring their survival in the changing health care and educational environment.

SUMMARY

The purpose of chapter 3 is to provide a conceptual framework for understanding marketing. Although it is often considered to be, marketing is not really a *new* activity for nursing organizations. What is perhaps new to most nursing organizations is the conduct of marketing activities as a series of interrelated events that are part of a strategic marketing process. The increasingly volatile nursing environment requires a comprehensive approach to marketing.

This chapter presents definitions of marketing, the marketing mix, the characteristics of nonprofit marketing, the relationship of strategic planning and strategic marketing, portfolio analysis, and a detailed description of the strategic marketing process. While this chapter focuses on marketing concepts, essential components, and presentation of the strategic marketing process, chapter 4 presents specific methods and techniques for implementing the strategic marketing process.

REFERENCES

Balint, J., Menninger, K., & Hurt, M. (1983). Job opportunities for master's prepared nurses. *Nursing Outlook, 31*(2), 109–114.

Barton, D. W., & Treadwell, D. R. (1978). Marketing: A synthesis of institutional soul-searching and aggressiveness. *New Directions for Higher Education, 21,* 77–84.

Department of Health and Human Services. (1982). *Nurse supply distribution and requirements. Third report to the congress.* Hyattsville, MD: DHHS.

Department of Health and Human Services. (1983). *The registered nurse population.* Washington, DC: U.S. Government Printing Office.

Enis, B. M. (1980). *Marketing principles.* Santa Monica, CA: Goodyear.

Gollattscheck, J. F. (1981). Caution! Marketing may be hazardous to your institutional health. In W. Keim & M. Keim (Eds.), *New directions for community colleges: Marketing the program* (pp. 99–105). San Francisco: Jossey-Bass.

Gulack, R. (1983, December). Why nurses leave nursing. *Registered Nurse,* 32–37.

Hauf, B. J. (1981). Nurse response to continuing education: Relevant factors in marketing success. *Journal of Continuing Education, 12*(5), 10–16.

Hillestad, S. G., & Berry, R. (1980). Applying strategic marketing. In *Hospital and Health Services Administration* (pp. 7–16).

Institute of Medicine. (1983). *Nursing and nursing education: Public policies and private actions.* Washington, DC: National Academy Press.

Kotler, P. (1980). *Marketing management, analysis, planning and control.* Englewood Cliffs, NJ: Prentice-Hall.

Kotler, P. (1982). *Marketing for nonprofit organizations.* Englewood Cliffs, NJ: Prentice-Hall.

Kotler, P., & Fox, K. (1985). *Strategic marketing for educational institutions.* Englewood Cliffs, NJ: Prentice-Hall.

Kotler, P., & Goldgehn, L. A. (1981). Marketing: A definition for community colleges. In W. Keim & M. Keim (Eds.), *New directions for community colleges: Marketing the program* (pp. 5–12). San Francisco: Jossey-Bass.

LaTour, S. A. (1984). Guest editorial: A plea for strategic marketing. *Journal of Health Care Marketing, 4*(4), 5–9.

Lewis, H. (1984, January). Part-time nursing: How much of a career? *Registered Nurse,* 34–37.

Lovelock, C. H. (1977). Concepts and strategies for health marketers, *Hospital and Health Services Administration, 22,* 50–62.

Lovelock, C. H., & Weinberg, C. B. (1978). Public and nonprofit marketing comes of age. In G. Zaltman & T. V. Bonoma (Eds.), *Review of marketing.* Chicago: American Marketing Association.

McCarthy, J. E. (1978). *Basic marketing.* Homewood, IL: Irwin.

McKenna, R. (1985). *The Regis Touch.* Reading, MA: Addison-Wesley.

Miaoulis, G., Anderson, D. C., LaPlaca, P. J., Geduldig, J. P., Giesle, R. H., & West, S. (1985). A model for hospital marketing decision processes and relationships. In P. D. Cooper (Ed.), *Health care markets: Issues and trends* (2nd ed., pp. 118–127). Rockville, MD: Aspen Systems Corporation.

National Commission Nursing. (1983). *Summary report and recommendations.* Chicago: American Hospital Association.

National League for Nursing. (1982). *Employment, mobility and personal characteristics of nurses newly licensed in 1980.* New York: National League for Nursing.

Pantages, T. J., & Creedon, C. F. (1978). Studies of college attrition 1950. 1975. *Review of Educational Research, 48*(1), 49–101.

Pride, W. M., & Ferrell, O. C. (1980). *Marketing basic concepts and decisions.* Englewood Cliffs, NJ: Prentice-Hall.

Ries, A., & Trout, J. (1986). *Marketing Warfare.* New York: McGraw-Hill.

Rothman, J., Teresa, J. G., Kay, T. L., Morningstar, G. C. (1983). *Marketing human service innovations.* Beverly Hills: Sage.

Stanton, W. J. (1978). *Fundamentals of marketing.* New York: McGraw-Hill.

Wise Yoder, P. S. (1981). Needs assessment as a marketing strategy. *Journal of Continuing Education, 12*(5), 18–23.

Zallocco, R. L., Joseph, W. B., & Doremus, H. (1984). Strategic market planning for hospitals. *Journal of Health Care Marketing, 4*(2), 19–28.

4

Operationalizing Strategic Marketing

Susan Bond Chambers

INTRODUCTION

The strategic-marketing process, like any administrative practice, is far simpler for an organization to conceptualize than to put into operation. Theoretically, marketing concepts and principles make "good administrative sense"; however, potential obstacles and the work necessary for success probably makes it impossible for a marketing function to be fully realized. Lack of preparation and planning can result in failure.

The first step for the administrator is to gain an understanding of marketing principles and concepts. The more strategies, techniques, and methods for marketing that an administrator has knowledge of, the better the administrator is able to market the organization successfully. This chapter provides information and examples useful in the implementation of the strategic-marketing process.

MARKETING THE MARKETING EFFORT

It is important to realize first that too many individuals in nursing organizations, at least initially, will view marketing as:

- Unethical—an activity that is beneath their professional standards.
- Threatening—something they have little knowledge about.

- Unnecessary—an activity that is a waste of their time.
- Not their job—an activity that does not concern them.

Even those individuals who support marketing will more often than not equate it with selling or promotion activities.

Since marketing is a change agent, personnel not only need to understand and appreciate the marketing concept and the strategic-marketing process, but they also need to be prepared to expect change within the organization. People can accept change more readily when they know it will occur and believe it has potential to be positive. Administrators too often take action without preparing the organization, something that results many times in personnel rebelling against the action. Hence, what was intended to have a positive effect on the organization results in stress and negative behavior (Gollattscheck, 1981).

While, ideally, an administrator would assume that personnel would support marketing for the "good of the organization," this is not always true. Hence, a useful strategy in explaining and gaining support for marketing activities is to detail their potential benefits. For example, if an objective of the marketing effort is to develop a national reputation for the nursing college, then a potential benefit for faculty members is the opportunity to develop a national reputation for themselves. Similarly, in a clinical setting, when the marketing effort is meant to attract more qualified, experienced staff nurses, the potential benefit to the head nurse is a more competent staff. Once personnel feel the marketing effort will benefit both the organization and themselves, they may be more willing to support the effort. The key in applying this strategy is to determine the needs and wants of the members of the organization and the ways a marketing effort might fulfill them.

A general rule in selling the marketing concept is this: the more communication, the better. Also, there are numerous avenues for communication. In a clinical setting, marketing can be communicated via departmental meetings, in-service activities, memorandums, bulletin boards, and agency publications (e.g., newsletters). One hospital's experience was that the nursing staff wanted everything written in concrete policies and had difficulty using flexibility; they found that the keys to success were involving the nursing staff in plans through unit and department meetings, providing general guidelines, and supplying in-service training (Armstrong et al., 1985).

In an educational setting, marketing can be explained via faculty assembly, department meetings, the school newsletter, in-service activities, memorandums, bulletin boards, and the school's board of visitor meetings.

In both clinical and educational settings, when one is attempting to teach what marketing is and isn't, care should be taken so that material is not presented in a patronizing manner. In addition, since marketing is an up-beat activity for the organization, presentations regarding marketing should be positive.

Informal communication must also not be forgotten. The more the nursing administrator talks about what is being done, the better. Informal communication also works two ways—that is, input, suggestions, guidance, and feedback should be sought on an informal basis.

No matter how well the marketing effort is presented, inevitably there will be members of the organization who are too threatened by marketing to ever support it, even if they have an understanding of the marketing concept. These members of the organization may have good reason to be threatened by marketing; that is, the strategic marketing process *does* seek to identify the strengths and weaknesses of the organization and those markets that are being best served. More specifically, for example, if faculty members are aware that their department is outdated and that students and others are not satisfied with their education, then they probably will be (and should be) threatened by marketing activities. On another dimension, it should be remembered that the strategic-marketing process *does* require a thorough audit of the organization's records. If the director of hospital admissions knows that records are not in order, potential requests for data may be threatening. In both of these cases, faculty and the admissions director will also probably demonstrate blocking behavior when marketing data is sought. Certainly, being aware of and expecting this behavior can be useful to the nursing administrator. The use of explicit Responsibility Charts and Gantt Charts (as advocated in chapter 3 and presented in chapter 6) are effective tools to help prevent this behavior, since responsibilities and activities of individuals at all levels of the organization are detailed. Responsibility and Gantt Charts also serve as additional avenues for communication.

Not only must the administrator market the marketing effort internally, but he or she also must market the marketing effort externally (i.e., to audiences outside the nursing organization). External communication is important in obtaining sources for marketing data and gaining acceptance for marketing activities among the local and health care communities, and nursing colleagues. A nursing college administrator needs to communicate marketing activities to the university administrators, and a hospital nursing department administrator needs to communicate marketing activities to the hospital administrators, since the support of the administrators above the nursing level can be especially valuable when funds are sought for marketing activities. Methods for accomplishing this in a clinical setting include newsletters, presentations at administrative meetings (e.g., department head meetings, board of trustees meeting), "marketing update" memorandums, and informal communication. In an educational setting, methods include presentations at administrative meetings (e.g., deans' meetings, university administrators' meetings, board of regents' meetings), university publications (e.g., newspapers, newsletters), "marketing update" memorandums, and informal communication.

Communicating marketing activities to the community can be accomplished through publicity efforts with local television, newspapers, and radio. Nursing is in a particularly advantageous position to obtain free publicity because of the shortage of nurses, the impact of nurses on the health of the community, and the uniqueness of applying marketing concepts in nursing organizations. Presentations to health care and educational associations, news releases to association newsletters, and informal communication regarding marketing practices and activities being conducted by the organization are also useful mechanisms to gain support for marketing data collection and other efforts.

A nursing administrator should realize, when publicizing the marketing effort, that he or she is also building expectations for the effort. Taking this into consideration, the administrator needs to be sure that marketing is not presented as a "cure-all" for the organization, and he or she must be committed to putting the marketing plan into effect. Building expectations and then shelving the marketing plan will have a disasterous impact upon the organization.

DESIGNING THE MARKETING ANALYSIS

Marketing analysis is the most important step of the strategic-marketing process. It is imperative that comprehensive, accurate, and valid data be collected upon which to base sound-marketing decisions. The steps of the strategic-marketing process that follow the marketing analysis are accomplished by utilizing the information collected during the analysis stage. The ability to link marketing plans and programs to objective data makes it easier to justify and defend marketing decisions.

As noted in chapter 3, the design of the marketing analysis is organized into three phases: organizational, market, and competitive (see Figure 1). The phases are not intended to be completed in a particular order and, in many instances, are best implemented concurrently. More specifically, there may be occasions at the data collection stage when it is more economical to collect information that addresses needs of all three phases. Consider the hospital record of a patient: It may provide information regarding what facilities of the hospital were utilized (organizational phase), what other agencies treated the patient in the past (competitive phase), and what future health needs the organization might be able to serve (market phase). It is more feasible to collect all of this information at once than to review the hospital admission record three separate times.

The data to be collected for a particular phase is guided by established information needs, which are questions related to the status of the organizational, competitive, and market environment of the nursing organization. These needs should be designed so that the data collected to address them is pertinent to marketing decisions.

Within each phase of the marketing analysis, it is useful if specific information needs are organized into similar content areas. Identification of content areas will help keep the marketing analysis focused. For example, a home health care agency might have areas of information needs in the organizational phase of personnel (nurses, clerical, and administrative), clients, financial, and service-related (i.e., information needs specific to the nursing services provided by the agency).

The number and specificity of information needs or questions should be determined on the basis of the stated goals and resources of the strategic marketing effort. However, the more specific the information needs are, the more specific the data collected will be, and the less likely is it that information will be collected that is not useful for marketing decision making.

In the design of the marketing analysis, consideration is also given to both present and future information needs (i.e., those that do not warrant immediate attention), since the strategic-marketing process is ongoing and needs to be proactive, rather than reactive. Furthermore, if more accurate record keeping results as an outcome of the marketing plan, future information needs will be considered when better record-keeping mechanisms are designed. The design of a marketing analysis is best explained via an example; that is, the design of a marketing analysis for a nursing school will be used for illustration purposes. Figure 1 depicts the design of a marketing analysis for a nursing school in which the levels of analysis consist of program levels and geographic area.

The Organizational Phase

The organizational phase involves an evaluation of the school as a provider of nursing education. The organizational phase is, in essence, an audit of the school's resources in order to identify the strengths and

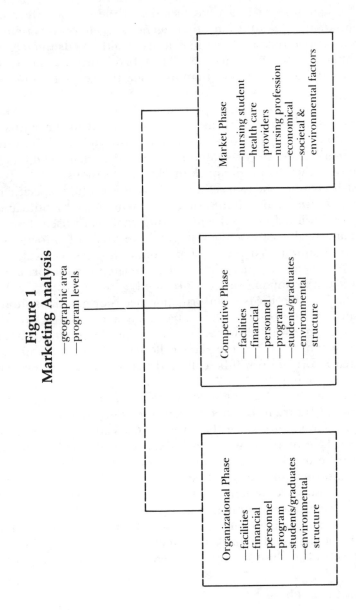

Figure 1
Marketing Analysis
—geographic area
—program levels

Organizational Phase

—facilities
—financial
—personnel
—program
—students/graduates
—environmental
structure

Competitive Phase

—facilities
—financial
—personnel
—program
—students/graduates
—environmental
structure

Market Phase

—nursing student
—health care
providers
—nursing profession
—economical
—societal &
environmental factors

weaknesses of the school. The information needs are organized into six areas, including:

1. Facilities—information needs related to adequacy (strengths and weaknesses) of existing facilities.
2. Financial—information needs related to financial aspects of the school of nursing (e.g., costs of programs, facilities, adequacy of funding, cost efficient resources).
3. Personnel—information needs related to needs and wants of personnel, outstanding personnel, factors that attract personnel.
4. Program—information needs related to characteristics of programs' curriculum, programs' reputations, programs' enrollment.
5. Students/graduates—information needs related to characteristics of students, factors that attract students, students' wants and needs.
6. Environmental structure—information needs related to locality of school, community relationship, university relationship.

Table 1 provides a sample of the type of information need appropriate for the area of facilities, i.e., "Of the facilities utilized by the school, which are a unique and/or outstanding resource or have the potential to be so?" Other information needs within the area of facilities might include:

Table 1
Marketing Analysis: Organizational Phase

Area	Information Need
1. Facilities	01.1 Of the facilities utilized by the school, which are a unique and/or outstanding resource or have the potential to be so?
2. Financial	02.1 What components (i.e., programs, services, personnel, departments, etc.) are most cost-efficient?
3. Personnel	03.1 Who in the school has a national, regional, and/or local reputation?
4. Program	04.1 What programs of the school are in demand as evidenced by enrollment data?
5. Students/graduates	05.1 What factors have attracted students to the school?
6. Environmental structure	06.1 How does the University setting contribute to the success of the school?

O1.2 Of the facilities (buildings, support services, clinical agencies), which are problematic (i.e., inadequate, costly)?

O1.3 What facilities are in demand by the school that are not available?

O1.4 What facilities does the school have available that are not utilized? underutilized? overutilized?

Each information need can be labeled, that is, the phase is abbreviated by the first letter (e.g., in the above example, organizational phase is O), the area of information needs is assigned a number (in the example, facilities was assigned "1"), and each information need is assigned the area number and another unique number (in the example, the first facilities information need was 1.1, the second, 1.2, and so on). Labeling each information need is useful for record-keeping purposes and saving time in data collection.

The levels of analysis concept is best illustrated by considering the information need O1.1, "Of the facilities utilized by the school, which are a unique and outstanding resource or have the potential to be so?" On an educational program level, facilities considered unique for the baccalaureate program may be very different than those for the doctoral program. Similarly, facilities considered unique on a local level for the baccalaureate program may be quite different than facilities considered unique on a national level.

The Competitive Phase

The competitive phase of the marketing analysis for a nursing school involves determining all competitors of the school, identifying their resources, and assessing their strengths and weaknesses. Competitors should be identified for each product offered. In this example, depending upon relevancy, competitors could be identified for each educational program and geographic level, that is, for the baccalaureate program on local, regional, and national levels; for the master's program, administration concentration on local and regional levels . . . and so on. Methods for identifying competitors in education include determining the following: schools students apply to; schools that offer similar educational programs; schools where faculty taught previously or where faculty accept new positions; schools that are ranked similarly; and schools that students, faculty, and administrators consider competitors.

Similarly, in health care agencies, competitors may be identified by determining the following: agencies offering similar services; agencies where nurses worked previously or where nurses accept new positions; agencies in which patients/clients have received similar services in the past; and agencies identified by the nursing staff and clients as competitors. Table 2 presents some potential data sources and methods for identifying competitors in education and clinical-nursing settings.

In order to enable comparison with the information gathered in the organizational phase, the competitive-phase information needs are organized into the same areas. In the example, this would include facilities, financial, personnel, program, students/graduates, and environmental structure. Specific competitive information needs appropriate for the nursing school are illustrated in Table 3.

The Market Phase

The market phase of the marketing analysis in education involves the assessment of current and potential opportunities and threats facing the market for nursing education. In the example, areas of information needs for the market phase are organized into:

1. Nursing student—information needs related to characteristics, preferences, supply, needs, expectations, and wants of nursing students.

2. Health care providers—information needs related to health care provider's demand, expectations, and needs for nurses.

3. Nursing profession—information needs related to the nursing profession's expectations of nursing education.

4. Economic, societal, and environmental—information needs related to the influence of economic, societal, and environmental factors on the provision of nursing education.

Specific information needs relevant to the market phase for this example are depicted in Table 4. As illustrated in Table 5, with minor modification, this marketing analysis design could be applied in a clinical setting. That is, in the organizational and competitive phase, the areas of information needs would be facilities, financial, personnel, nursing interventions offered, patients/clients, and environmental structure. The market phase would be organized into patient/client, health care profession, nursing profession, and economic and societal factors.

Table 2
Data Sources for Identifying Competitors

Educational		Clinical	
Data to be Identified	**Source**	**Data to be Identified**	**Source**
Other schools students/applicants submit applications to	Student application, exit interviews	Other agencies patients/clients have received similar services	Admitting forms
Schools that offer similar programs	NLN listing of accredited programs, library, brochures	Agencies that offer similar services	Health care associations, state, and federal agencies
Schools faculty transfer to or come from	Faculty vitae, exit interviews	Agencies nurses transfer to or come from	Position applications, exit interviews
Schools that are ranked similarly	Educational literature, nursing literature	Agencies identified by staff as competitors	Formal or informal survey of staff (e.g., at department meetings)
Schools considered competitors by faculty and administrators	Formal or informal survey of faculty and administrators (e.g., at department meetings, faculty assembly)		

Table 3
Marketing Analysis: Competitive Phase

Area	Information Need
1. Facilities	What facilities (i.e., campus buildings, clinical agencies, support services, etc.) does the competitor have?
2. Financial	What does the competitor currently charge for tuition?
3. Personnel	Does the competitor have certain people in the school who are a unique and outstanding resource?
4. Program	Does the competitor's program attract students of a higher caliber than similar programs?
5. Students/graduates	What are the student recruitment efforts of the competitor?
6. Environmental structure	How does the location of the competitor contribute to the success of the school?

When the marketing information system is being established, it is important to obtain as much input from individuals in the organization as possible. Viewpoints from a variety of perspectives will help to keep the analysis comprehensive and valid. One can accomplish this by first constructing a draft of suggested information needs and then circulating this draft throughout the organization. This technique is recommended, since the draft gives individuals an idea of what is expected as far as input and also serves as an additional communication tool.

While the design of the marketing analysis presented here may be far too elaborate for some nursing organizations, the content and principles suggested are relevant as a general guideline. That is, even in

Table 4
Marketing Analysis: Market Phase

Area	Information Need
1. The nursing student	What are the needs (e.g., educational, personal, and environmental) of the nursing student?
2. Health care providers	In what role areas do health care providers identify an actual or potential demand for nurses?
3. The nursing profession	What changes in nursing education does the nursing profession propose in order to enhance the image and quality of professional nursing?
4. Economic, societal, and environmental factors	Given the changing health care environment, what are society's expectations from nursing education and practice?

Table 5
Marketing Analysis Design

Organizational Phase		Competitive Phase		Market Phase	
Education	Service	Education	Service	Education	Service
Facilities	Facilities	Facilities	Facilities	The nursing student	Patients/clients
Financial	Financial	Financial	Financial	Health care providers	The health care profession
Personnel	Personnel	Personnel	Personnel	The nursing profession	The nursing profession
Program	Nursing intervention offered	Program	Nursing intervention offered	Economical, societal, environmental factors	Economical and societal factors
Students/graduates	Patients/clients	Students/graduates	Patients/clients		
Environmental structure	Environmental structure	Environmental structure	Environmental structure		

smaller organizations, it is necessary to consider what the organizational strengths and weaknesses are, what the competitor's strengths and weaknesses are, and what market opportunities and threats exist before the organization can make marketing decisions.

IDENTIFYING SECONDARY DATA SOURCES

The first step in attempting to address information needs is to identify, collect, and review available secondary data. One useful strategy for identifying data sources is to include a column when one is establishing the marketing analysis information needs, entitled "Potential Data Sources." Doing this will enable the brainstorming of data sources as information needs are identified. As an example, consider the following organizational information need and potential data sources:

Organizational (O)
Student/Graduate (5)

Information Need	*Potential Data Sources*
05.1 What do students/graduates feel are the strengths of the school?	Alumni survey
	Program assessment questionnaire
	Course evaluation questionnaire
	Evaluation of continuing education offerings
	Exit interviews

Providing this type of format facilitates the brainstorming necessary to identify existing data sources. The potential data sources can be solicited at the same time input to what information needs should be included in the marketing analysis is solicited.

There is an abundance of documentation available in nursing organizations, the usefulness of which is never fully realized. The marketing analysis provides for the synthesis of this collective information for use in making strategic-marketing decisions. Some of the useful internal documentation available in nursing education organizations includes the following: annual reports, committee minutes and reports, faculty vitae, budgets, financial reports, accreditation reports, enrollment statistics, grant proposals, and all reports emanating from evaluation activities. In nursing service organizations, documents with potential use for the marketing analysis include the following: performance evaluations, quality assurance activities, annual reports, admissions statistics, budget/income statements, committee minutes, employment applications, agency records, agency brochures, agency newsletters, and certificate-of-need reports.

Competitive information in nursing service may be available from state agency studies, competitor's advertisements in newspapers and television, competitor's brochures, and newspaper articles. The primary sources in nursing education for competitive information are the nursing education brochures and catalogs. Other sources include journal and newspaper articles and advertisements, as well as school newsletters.

For the market analysis, there is an abundance of information via national, regional, and state organizations. Nursing literature is also rich in studies that provide information regarding market trends. A strategy for obtaining sources for market information is to request information from health care associations, federal and state agencies, and other potential sources. The response in both quantity and quality of information, and in the level of interest and cooperation from these organizations, will quite often be surprising. This technique costs very little and is "good press" for the organization, i.e., communicates that the organization is implementing a comprehensive marketing effort and is genuinely interested in meeting market needs. In addition to the nursing literature, the following provides a sample of potential market information sources:

- Private foundations
- State agency publications (planning, vital statistics)
- National nursing organizations
- National health care associations
- State nursing associations
- State health care associations
- Chambers of commerce
- Local government agencies
- Local and national newspapers
- Proceedings of conferences
- Special interest health care groups
- Special interest nursing societies

- Federal agencies
- Consulting companies
- Private foundations
- Published rankings

EXHAUSTING THE USEFULNESS OF SECONDARY DATA

More extensive analysis of existing data can enhance its meaning. For example, in an educational environment, enrollment statistics and financial data can be compared to determine a cost per full time equivalent (FTE) student by educational program or even by concentration within a program. If all financial data is not retrievable by program, faculty and staff salaries are a good determinant of cost and are easily retrievable. In addition, enrollment statistics can be put into better perspective if calculations are made for:

- Percentage increase or decrease in FTE students over time by program/concentration.
- Percentage contribution of program/concentration to total enrollment.
- Percentage part-time status versus full-time status by program/concentration over time.
- Percentage enrollment by program/concentration by geographical area over time.
- Percentage enrollment of higher test scores and grade point average (GPA) scores by program/concentration.
- Percentage increase or decrease in average GPA and test scores over time.
- Percentage enrollment by prior years of nursing experience over time.

Combinations of calculations of the above can also be useful. For example, determining if students from a specific geographic area are more likely to attend full-time or part-time would be useful information for identifying target markets.

Content analysis of faculty vitae is another useful way to obtain more information from existing data. For example, the following may be extracted from faculty vitae: highest degree and degree area of specialization, number of honors, number of publications (articles, books, etc.), number of years' experience teaching in particular specialties, number of community activities, program/concentration currently teaching in, geographic location of residence, and so forth. This information can be entered on the computer to enable cross-tabulation analysis to determine, for example, the concentration in which faculty have been most active in publishing.

In a clinical setting, admission records of patients can be analyzed to determinc:

- Number of patients by admission diagnosis.

- Average length of stay by diagnosis.

- Profile (geographic, age, income, etc.) of patients by diagnosis.

- Number of ancilliary procedures by diagnosis.

Admission records can be paired with costs to determine information such as nursing cost per patient by diagnosis.

In the clinical setting, evaluations of nursing personnel can be content-analyzed to determine, for example, what nurses' performance level is by department, what weaknesses and strengths in nursing personnel are universal or generalizable, and what the characteristics are of nurses on staff who perform exceptionally well (e.g., demographic information).

In either a nursing clinical or educational setting, content-analyzing competitors' advertisements can be an effective method to gain marketing information. More specifically, a standard form is filled out for each advertisement and may include such items as the following: what market(s) is the competitor targeting? What offering(s) is the competitor promoting? What differential advantage(s) is the competitor promoting? What advertising medium is the competitor using? Using a standard form ensures the same information is being collected for all competitors.

The preceding material illustrates a few ways to exhaust the meaningfulness of existing data. Obviously, these techniques are preferable to collecting new data for reasons of efficiency. It should be kept in mind that even though secondary data is valuable, it only tells you what is happening, not why it is happening (Gaither, 1980).

ORGANIZING SECONDARY DATA

When one reviews and collects secondary data, it is helpful for record-keeping purposes to (1) organize the information in accordance with the design of the marketing analysis, and (2) to assign each refer-

Table 6
Sample of Format for Collecting Marketing Information

Source	Information	Level of Analysis	Information Need Addressed
1	The majority of the 1987 baccalaureate-RN graduates rated "the extent to which library facilities are adequate" as 4 (agree strongly) on a scale of 1 (disagree strongly) to 4 (agree strongly)	3	01.1
90	The library is ranked as one of the top 10 of health science libraries across the nation	8	01.1

ence source a number. More specifically, consider Table 6, which illustrates a format for collecting secondary data. The first source listed is denoted as "1," which is identified in a source listing as the "1987 Report of the Program Assessment Questionnaire Results." The "3" under level of analysis signifies "Baccalaureate RN program, all geographic levels." The information need addressed is O1.1, "Of the facilities of the school which are a unique and outstanding resource or have the potential to be so?" With the use of a word processor, it is easy to see that a system such as this one helps to keep the data collection organized. With the addition of a computer program, information could be sorted by source, information need addressed, and level of analysis.

CONDUCTING PRIMARY DATA ANALYSIS

Most nursing organizations, despite the abundance of secondary data sources, will need to conduct marketing-research activities to collect data that is specific to critical information needs. Once secondary-data sources are exhausted, those information needs that are not adequately addressed and that are deemed vital to developing marketing strategies are identified. Marketing research is then designed to address these information needs. Viewed in this light, the marketing information needs facilitate keeping primary data analysis focused because marketing research is designed to address specific questions, and time is not wasted collecting information that would just be "nice to know." Types of information not likely to be provided by secondary data sources in a nursing clinic environment, as an example, may include:

Why do patients choose our clinic over others?

What is the image of the clinic as perceived by the community?

Why do employees (nurses, secretaries, technicians, etc.) choose to work here?

In an educational environment, the type of information not addressed by secondary sources would probably include:

What influences our benefactors and alumni to donate to the nursing college?

What attracts students to the nursing college?

What do faculty see as the greatest weakness of the nursing college?

In addition to providing marketing information, conducting marketing research also communicates to those whose involvement is requested that the organization is genuinely interested in meeting consumer needs. In this way, there is a positive side effect or additional advantage to conducting marketing research.

Conducting this type of research in a nursing organization is not very different than conducting any other research. The purposes for the research and the need for it to be conducted in an efficient manner are, as one would expect, different. A couple of useful, efficient methods and strategies for generating primary data in both nursing clinical and educational settings include, but certainly are not limited to, the following:

- Telephone logs
- Addendums to evaluation forms
- Addendums to current record-keeping practices
- Recruitment reporting forms
- Linking survey administration with other procedures
- Computer mapping
- Focus groups
- Interviews

A telephone log is a listing of complaints, inquiries, questions, and recommendations received by phone. When a telephone log is established, it is necessary that all departments that deal with the public are keeping the log in the same manner. The log provides an objective means to quantify compliments, complaints, and inquires related to particular products. Information solicited on a telephone log might include date of call, caller's name, caller's reference group (e.g., patient or student, previous patient or alumni, community member), subject matter of call (e.g., parking, master's program curriculum, emergency room), nature of call (e.g., complaint, compliment, information inquiry), and specific topic. Table 7 is a sample telephone log for the nursing department of a hospital.

Adding an addendum to evaluation forms is an efficient method to collect marketing information, and it saves time and money in terms of both data collection and analysis. As an example of use of an addendum, an evaluation form for a workshop may have additional questions such as: What other workshops would you like offered? What inspired you to attend this workshop? Why did you choose this workshop over XYZ's workshop? How did you learn of this workshop?

In the clinical setting, an addendum of nonthreatening questions may be part of a nurse's evaluation, for example: How do you feel more patients could be attracted to the hospital? Who do you feel are competitors of the hospital? How do you think the community views the hospital?

Similar to adding an addendum to evaluation forms is adding marketing questions to current record-keeping practices. There are numerous opportunities to apply this strategy; in the clinical setting, consider:

• Inserting a patient satisfaction survey with the bill for services. The patient can complete the survey and return it with payment of the bill, hence, there is no additional mailing cost involved.

• Adding marketing questions to the admitting forms completed by patients. Questions might include: Why did you choose the hospital to serve your health care needs? What other hospitals were considered? On a scale of 1 (not at all) to 6 (to a great extent), how important were the following in your selection:

> location of hospital____;
>
> reputation for excellence____;
>
> cleanliness of hospital____;
>
> physician chose this hospital____;
>
> physician recommended this hospital____.

• Adding marketing questions to the nurses' job application form. Questions include: What are the three most important factors to you in your job selection? Why did you choose to apply for a job at this hospital? What job benefits are most important to you?

Table 7
Telephone Log for the Nursing Department of XYZ Hospital

Date	Caller	Reference Group	Subject Matter	Nature of Call	Specific Topic
8/1	John Doe	Patient's family	Parking	Complaint	Mr. Doe was unable to park in hospital parking lot from 7/10–7/21
8/2	Mary Smith	Previous patient	Nurse performance in OB/GYN	Compliment	Mrs. Smith wanted supervisor to know that Nurse Brown provided her with excellent care

In a nursing educational environment, an addendum can be included with existing record-keeping practices in the following ways:

- Marketing questions can be added to student application forms. Questions include: How did you first become aware of the school? What other schools have you applied to? What factors are influential in your selection of a school?

- The pledge cards for fund raising can include marketing questions. For example, questions may include: What do you see as the strengths of the school? weaknesses? What types of alumni activities would you like to see offered?

- Marketing questions can be added to the registration form for a conference. Questions may include: Why did you elect to attend this conference? What do you perceive to be the greatest strength of our school? weakness? What topic areas would you like to see included in future offerings?

To ascertain recruitment information, a useful strategy is to design a reporting form that the recruiter fills out. In an educational environment, Larkin (1980) suggests that the form include such items as the following: (1) What did you see that suggests student needs? (2) What led you here? (3) What did you make of your observations? Similarly, a nurse recruiter may complete a form that includes essentially the same information, that is: (1) What did you see that suggest nurse needs? (2) What led you here? (3) What did you make of your observations?

In order to administer surveys with as much ease as possible, one can include them with other routine activities/practices. As an example, in both clinical and educational settings, personnel can be given a survey to complete when they receive their paychecks. In a clinical environment, a patient satisfaction survey might be administered as part of the departure procedures of the hospital. Students may be requested to complete a marketing survey as part of graduation materials.

Computer mapping is a useful technique in both nursing clinical and educational environments, providing a visual method of depicting the geographic distribution of a group of people (Gaither, 1980). Such mapping in an educational environment could provide the geographical distribution of students and include geographical spread by program, concentration, full-time/part-time status, and so forth. In a clinical environment, computer mapping could illustrate geographic distribution of patients and include geographic spread by diagnosis, insurance, and coverage. Computer mapping could also be used to depict where employees (faculty, nurses, etc.) live. Some of the existing programs available include Synagraphic Computer Mapping (SYMAP) and Choropletter Mapping (CORMAP).

Focus groups are simply a small group (5–15 members) who are guided in an informal discussion; members should be comprised of people who are comfortable with one another. The discussion should be guided in a loose, nonthreatening manner. Focus groups are useful in brainstorming a wide variety of ideas, problems, and issues. As an example, focus groups of students may be asked to address questions such as the following: What led you to decide to be a nurse? What factors were most influential in your selection of this school? What are your most important educational needs? How would you describe the image of this school? What (if any) personal needs do you feel the school needs to consider? A focus group of nurses may be asked such questions as the following: What is the most desirable aspect of your job? How could the clinic better meet your professional needs? What would cause you to leave your job? How do you think the needs of patients could better be met?

Interviews can be an effective method to obtain marketing information. In organizations, personnel often are the best source of information regarding history of the organization, interpersonal issues, environment of the organization, and why certain practices have been successful and others have not. Questionnaires do not always provide personnel with enough prodding or coaching to share the full extent of their knowledge about the organization, however. In addition, interviews must be conducted by a nonthreatening individual, who may even need to be an outside consultant. Anonymity of the interviewee should be assured.

REPORTING MARKETING RESEARCH RESULTS

A clear, concise report of results of marketing research is as important as the methodology employed. The report should include the following content:

1. Purpose—a brief statement of, in general terms, what marketing information was being sought.
2. Sample or respondents—a description of who was responding to the survey instrument.
3. Methodology—a summary of what marketing information needs

were addressed, how the research was designed, and how data was collected and analyzed.

4. Results—included in the results section are response rates, reliability and validity statistics, and results as they relate to each marketing information need and each level of analysis. By organizing the results according to marketing information need and level of analysis, results are easily incorporated with other marketing information for a particular information need. For example, suppose an applicant survey addressed the information need, "Why do students choose to attend this college?" Results for this question would be reported for all students, for baccalaureate students, for baccalaureate students from out of state, etc.

5. Appendices—included should be tables of all results and a copy of the data collection instrument.

Several key points are worth remembering when one is writing marketing research reports:

1. Keep the report short and concise. Lengthy reports tend to lose the reader's interest.

2. Write the report assuming the reader has no knowledge of the marketing effort. Reports are often widely disseminated, and readers require sufficient background to understand results.

3. Include only basic statistics and use nontechnical language. Advanced statistics are only understood and appreciated by researchers; most readers have no use for them.

4. Include tables of all results. This will provide the reader results for any item that may not have been addressed in the body of the report.

5. Be sure every statement made is backed up by data. This keeps the report objective and factual.

SYNTHESIZING MARKETING DATA TO DETERMINE MARKETING OPPORTUNITIES AND THREATS

Once the administrator has collected, exhausted, analyzed, and collated the marketing data, the potential to become overwhelmed by the information is great. Organizing the data by information needs, as suggested previously, helps to keep the synthesis manageable.

A recommended procedure for synthesizing the data is the following:

1. Read through the information collected several times.
2. Identify those findings or themes that seem to be repetitive.
3. Read through the data again and keep a tally of the amount of times themes are repeated and also the source which cites this finding or theme.
4. Using the tally, construct a list of (a) market opportunities and threats, (b) competitor strengths and weaknesses, and (c) organizational strengths and weaknesses.
5. If the list becomes too lengthy to be meaningful, eliminate those items not as strongly verified in the data.
6. At least one other individual should do 1–5 above; results are compared and discussed until concensus is reached.

On the basis of the three lists, major marketing opportunities and threats should evolve. As an example, suppose the following findings resulted for a nursing school:

Organizational Strength

Faculty, students, alumni, and the nursing profession view the school of nursing as a leader and innovator in providing nursing education.

Market Opportunity

The home health care market is expanding at a rapid rate, and the demand for nurses with advanced preparation in home health care has exceeded the supply locally, regionally, and nationally.

Competitor Strength

XYZ School of Nursing offers a baccalaureate program that has a specialty in home health care.

From these three findings, a marketing opportunity may be for the school to develop and offer a concentration (master's degree) in home health care. This opportunity would have evolved, given that the competition offers a home health care specialty at the baccalaureate level (not the master's level), there is a growing demand for nurses at this level, and the school has a reputation of being innovative.

Consider the following findings for a nurse clinic:

Organizational Weakness

Nurse applicants and patients have expressed concern regarding the location of the clinic in a high-crime area.

Market Threat

Potential clients identify the location of the clinic as the primary reason why they would choose to not come to the clinic.

Competitive Strength

XYZ Clinic is only 10 minutes from the clinic and is in a more desirable area.

Obviously, from this information, a marketing threat would be the location of the clinic in a high-crime area.

SEGMENTING MARKETS

Numerous variables can be considered when one segments markets for educational and clinical nursing products. Table 8 lists some of the variables that may be considered. Segmenting a market is simply a trial-and-error procedure until the most meaningful and useful segmentation is identified.

Demographic and psychographic variables are the two most commonly used categories for segmentation. Demographic variables are characteristics of individuals such as age, sex, and occupation. Psychographic variables are characteristics of individuals such as social class (e.g., low, middle, upper-middle), lifestyle (e.g., jet-setter, yuppie, conservative), personality traits (e.g., aggressive, passive, innovator, risk-taker), and specific buyer characteristics (e.g., benefits sought, buyer patterns).

As one might expect, demographic segmentation is much more easily accomplished than psychographic segmentation. This is due mainly to the prevalence of demographic data available from secondary sources

Table 8
Variables for Consideration in Market Segmentation in Nursing

Demographic
  Sex
  Age
  Stage in family life cycle (e.g., single, married/no children, married w/one child,
    divorced, etc.)
  Education level
  Occupation
  Position title (e.g., head nurse, staff nurse, etc.)
  Employer Characteristics (e.g., state hospital, VA hospital, private nursing home, etc.)
  Geographic location of residence (e.g., state, county, city, rural, urban, suburban)
  Geographic location of employer
  Income level
  Job experience
  Race
  Religion
  Nationality

Psychographic
  Social class (low, low-middle, upper-middle, etc.)
  Lifestyle (jetsetter, conservative, etc.)
  Benefits sought (prestige, knowledge, better position)
  Personality traits (risktaker, innovative, passive, aggressive, etc.)

(e.g., census bureau, state agencies, health care associations). Demographic information is also collected frequently in day-to-day internal record-keeping practices (e.g., application forms, personnel records, patient records, evaluation forms).

Obviously, in order to segment a market, data needs to be collected regarding relevant demographic and psychographic variables. More specifically, at the time primary data collection questionnaires are designed, potentially relevant segmentation variables should be identified and included on the questionnaire. Subsequently, if there are market differences, that is, differences in needs and wants regarding the nursing products offered, they can be identified.

Most nursing administrators have a general idea of relevant segmentation variables. For example, most nursing education administrators know that a few of the following influence students' needs and wants regarding nursing education: age, nursing experience, full-time/part-time working status, income, previous education, location of residence and/or employer, and career aspirations. What the education nurse administrator does not know is which of these variables, or which combination of variables, result in the strongest market segments.

DEVELOPING MARKETING STRATEGIES— SELECTING TARGET MARKETS

As chapter 3 describes, the marketing opportunities and threats provide the basis for determining the marketing objectives and goals, as well as concurrently developing marketing strategies. Every objective and goal should relate to a marketing opportunity or threat. By the relating of each objective and goal to a marketing opportunity or threat, another mechanism is put in place to ensure that the marketing plan is data based.

Marketing strategy is the selection of a target market(s), the choice of a competitive position, and the development of an effective marketing mix to reach and serve the chosen market (Kotler, 1982). As one can surmise, the first step in developing a marketing strategy is to select a target market(s). In addition to consideration of the attractiveness of the market, the nursing administrator must simultaneously consider its organizational strengths and weaknesses and the competitors' strengths and weaknesses relative to the market(s).

Once the most meaningful market segmentation has been accomplished, a useful strategy for choosing a target market(s) is to consider the possible patterns of coverage. With this approach, the nursing organization can decide whether it wants to offer one product to all markets, one product to a specific combination of markets, or one product to one market.

More specifically, Kotler (1982) suggests there are five general patterns of coverage available to an organization. Figures 2 and 3 illustrate segmentation of the nursing administration product market and the five patterns of coverage for a master's in nursing administration program, respectively.

The market for the master's in nursing administration program was segmented on the basis of nursing experience, that is, the markets were segmented into:

1. Nurses with only one to three years of nursing experience.
2. Nurses with 5–10 years of nursing experience.
3. Nurses who have executive administrative experience.

The products that the nursing school determined it could offer these markets consists of a master's in nursing administration program that has:

1. An administration in nursing homes emphasis.

Figure 2
Segmentation of the Nursing Administration Product Market

NURSING ADMINISTRATION PRODUCTS		MARKETS: Nurses with 1–3 years experience	Nurses with 5–10 years experience	Nurses with executive administrative experience
	Nursing Homes Emphasis			
	Hospital Emphasis			
	Home Health Care Emphasis			

Adapted with permission from Kotler, P. (1982). *Marketing for nonprofit organizations* (2nd Ed.), Englewood Cliffs, NJ: Prentice Hall Inc., p. 104.

Figure 3
Five Patterns of Market Coverage

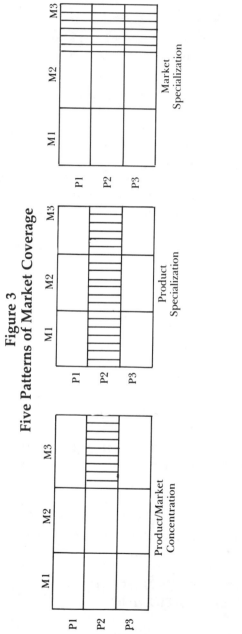

Product/Market
Concentration

Product
Specialization

Market
Specialization

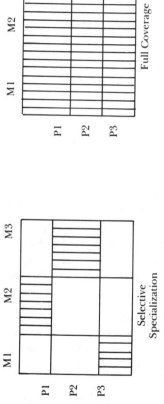

Full Coverage

Selective
Specialization

Adapted with permission from Abell D. F. (1980). *Defining the business: The starting point of strategic planning.* Englewood Cliffs, NJ: Prentice-Hall Inc., pp. 191–214.

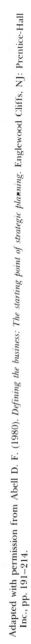

2. An administration in hospital emphasis.

3. An administration in home health care emphasis.

The five patterns of coverage available for the master's in nursing administration program, as suggested by Kotler (1982) and illustrated in Figure 4, include the following:

1. *Product/market concentration*—the offering of one product to one market segment. In the example, product/market concentration would be to offer a master's of nursing administration with a hospital emphasis to the executive nurse market segment.

2. *Product specialization*—the offering of one product to all market segments. In the example, product specialization would be to offer a master's of nursing administration with a hospital emphasis to all of the market segments, that is, nurses with all different types of experience.

3. *Market specialization*—the offering of all products to one market segment. In the example, market specialization would be to offer all three emphases in nursing administration to nurses who have executive experience.

4. *Selective specialization*—offering various products to various market segments that have no relationship to each other except that they individually represent a good marketing opportunity. In the example, selective specialization would be to offer a master's in nursing administration with (a) nursing home emphasis to nurses with 5–10 years of experience, (b) hospital emphasis to nurses with executive experience, and (c) home health care emphasis to nurses with only one to three years of nursing experience.

5. *Full coverage*—offering all products to all market segments. In the example, full coverage would be to offer all three emphases to all three market segments.

Of course, reality is not always as clearcut as this example appears to be. However, use of Kotler's framework is helpful in the sense that the model enables the nurse administrator to consider the options in a structured manner.

DEVELOPING MARKETING STRATEGIES— COMPETITIVE POSITIONING

When selecting which market(s) to serve, the nursing organization needs to consider a competitive positioning strategy, that is, what offer to make in relation to competitors' offerings. As exemplified in Figure 4, it can be useful to depict competitors' positions relative to their offering(s) to the market segments. Suppose, as illustrated in the figure, XYZ neighboring nursing school offers a master's in nursing administration with a hospital emphasis for nurses with varying levels of experience, ABC Nursing College offers a master's in nursing administration with all three emphases to nurses with all levels of experience, and DEF Nursing Department offers a master's in nursing administration with a nursing home and a hospital emphasis to nurses with all levels of experience. Given this information and that there is sufficient demand and organizational resources, the school may want to offer a master's in nursing administration (with all three emphasis) to only nurses who have executive experience.

As mentioned in chapter 3, another method to facilitate developing a competitive positioning strategy is to analyze the portfolios of competitors using the General Electric (GE) Portfolio grid technique.

DEVELOPING MARKETING STRATEGIES— DETERMINING THE MARKETING MIX

Obviously, the target market selected and the competitive positioning strategy chosen influence the development of the marketing mix. As defined previously, the marketing mix is composed of price, promotion, place, and product variables.

Consider the example, used previously, of the school that chose to offer a master's in nursing administration to executive nurses. The product is something that will fulfill the executive nurses' need for a master's education in nursing administration. The product, or content of the education program, is dictated by the level of experience, the learning characteristics, and the preferences for content of this target market.

Similarly, the price variable needs to be:

1. Appropriate for the target market.
2. At a level to cover costs of providing the product.
3. Considerate of the opportunity, effort, and psychic costs.
4. Congruent with the image of the product.

When the tuition for the master's in administration for nurse executives programs is established, it is probable that a higher tuition than competitors is appropriate, since:

Figure 4
Competitor Positions in the Master's in Nursing Administration Product Market

	Nurses with 1–3 years experience	Nurses with 5–10 years experience	Nurses with executive administrative experience
Nursing Home Emphasis	A D	A D	A D
Hospital Emphasis	A X D	A X D	A X D
Home Health Care Emphasis	A	A	A

X = XYZ Nursing School

A = ABC Nursing College

D = DEF Nursing Department

1. The target market can afford a higher tuition.
2. The higher tuition will pay for the cost of providing the program.
3. The opportunity, effort, and psychic costs of the program to executive nurses will be higher, hence, special arrangements (e.g., flexible scheduling, independent study, etc.) will need to be made that add additional cost to the program.
4. The specialized nature of the program denotes a higher quality, and a higher quality denotes a higher price.

Place variables are influenced by the target market needs and characteristics. These variables in the example include decisions about making the master's in nursing administration program accessible to the executive nurses. Given the hectic schedules of the executive nurse target market, it can be assumed that provisions may need to be made to offer weekend programs, study at home options, and/or to relocate classes to a more convenient proximity.

Promotion strategies are influenced by characteristics of the target market. Obviously, promotion strategies are developed after the product, place, and price variables are decided upon, and these variables influence the development of the promotion variable. For the master's in nursing administration program for executive nurses, which offers specialized content, flexible scheduling, and high cost of tuition, promotional activities need to convey these characteristics. More specifically, because these characteristics represent an elitist-type program, promotion strategies need to convey this image, as well. These may include sponsoring an "invitation only" reception to introduce the program and developing an advertising theme that expresses a "for executives only" approach.

DEVELOPING MARKETING STRATEGIES— THE PRODUCT LIFE-CYCLE

All products can be viewed as being in a stage of a life cycle. The product life cycle concept derives from the fact that a product's sales volume (or volume of benefits) follows a typical pattern (Clifford, 1980). As depicted in Figure 5, the product life cycle consists of four stages—introduction, growth, maturity, and decline (obsolescence). The length of each stage, actual shape of the curve, and length of the entire life cycle vary for different products. The profit or return on a

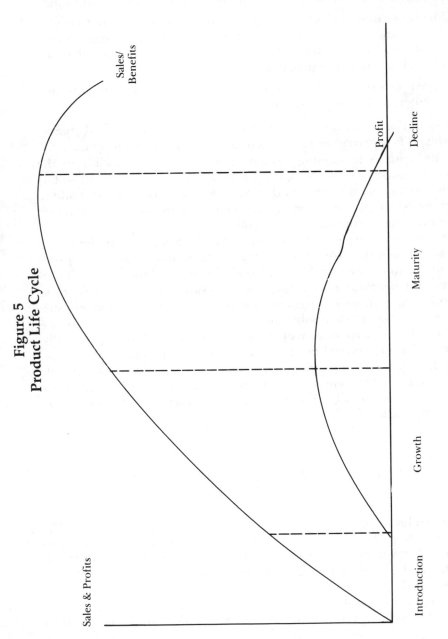

**Figure 5
Product Life Cycle**

product is at a different level for each stage. Likewise, the marketing strategies appropriate vary for each stage.

Introduction

Introduction is typically characterized by a low sales volume (or benefit volume) and negative profit or return on investment. The negative profit is due to the high initial costs of distribution and promotion. During the introduction stage, marketing strategy focuses on product development and design. Promotion strategies are directed toward acceptance of a new idea. In nursing, examples of products in the introduction stage include:

- The services of the nurse practitioner in roles more traditionally performed by physicians.
- The idea of the existence of two levels of nursing—professional and technical.
- The idea of the doctoral degree as the minimum educational requirement for nurse faculty.

Growth

Growth is the stage of soaring sales volume (or benefit volume) and profit or return on investment levels. While competitors begin to become more prevalent, there are still few of them. Acceptance has been achieved; therefore, the market for the product has expanded.

Marketing strategies in the growth stage are directed toward maintaining product quality. In order to sustain rapid growth, new markets and product features must be sought. Nursing products in the growth stage include:

- The service of providing home health care nursing and home health care nursing education.
- The service of providing gerontological nursing services and gerontological nursing education.
- The idea of applying strategic marketing principles in nursing education and service.

Maturity

Maturity is characterized by the peak and tapering off of sales volume and profit levels. Most products are in the maturity stage. At maturity, more competitors have entered the market, and competition is intensified. Marketing strategies are focused on product differentiation, locating new markets, and/or competitive pricing and distribution. Of course, there are numerous nursing products in the stage of maturity, including:

- The service of providing generic baccalaureate nursing education.
- The service of primary nursing in hospitals.
- The service of providing a master's in nursing with a clinical specialization emphasis.

Decline

Decline is the least desired stage of the product life cycle and is characterized by rapidly declining sales (or acceptance of benefits) and profits (or return). The decline stage can last a long or short time, depending upon the product. Typically, competitors leave the market at the decline stage. Those that remain in the market might be able to sustain, given the limited competition. Marketing strategies during the decline stage include the following: reduce product offerings, concentrate on the largest market segments, reduce distribution channels, reduce the promotion budget, and determine the best time to stop providing the product. Nursing products in the decline stage include the service of providing a diploma program education and the idea of a nurse as subservient to the physician.

DEVELOPING MARKETING STRATEGIES— A CONSUMER DECISION MODEL

The goal of the promotion variable of the marketing mix is to communicate effectively with markets; it is more appropriately called the communication variable. To determine the best approach or strategy for communicating to markets, it is expedient to consider the consumer's stage of decision making. MacStravic (1985), in his book entitled *Managing Health Care Marketing Communication*, presents a Consumer Decision Model that is applicable to most situations and is useful for understanding and influencing behavior. By identifying the stage of decision making of the target consumer, the nursing administrator can communicate information that is appropriate for the consumer's information-seeking needs. The model consists of six stages of consumer decision making:

1. *Problem recognition*—acknowledgment of a need.
2. *Application of existing knowledge*—consideration of what the individual already knows.
3. *Search for new information*—attempt to locate new information.
4. *Evaluation of alternatives*—comparison of new and existing information.
5. *Selection of an alternative*—decision on a provider.
6. *Implementation of selection*—act of consuming a product.

In each stage of behavior, different types of communication or communication strategy are recommended. The types of appropriate communication are best illustrated through an example. Consider the consumer with a heart problem. Suppose a center for heart diseases believes the high incidence of fatal heart attacks in the community is due to lack of early detection. Communication strategies would be directed toward (1) stimulation for consumers to recognize their heart problems and (2) information regarding symptoms.

If the center for heart diseases believes that not enough of the general public know of its existence, their communication is focused at the application of existing knowledge. Mass coverage of the existence of and general information about the center for heart diseases becomes the communication strategy. In other words, this type of communication ensures that an individual already has knowledge of the organization before feeling the need for the organization's products.

When the consumer is searching for information regarding his or her condition and the appropriate way to deal with it, communication focuses on the likelihood that the consumer will find such information. In the case of a consumer at the point of searching for a facility to provide care for his or her heart problem, it becomes important that communication about the center for heart diseases is accessible. This may be accomplished, for example, through communication with general practitioner physicians.

When the target consumer is at the stage of evaluation of alternatives, communication needs to take into consideration individual values. For example, the center for heart diseases needs to consider what is important to the heart patient when he or she selects a facility. Factors such as educational preparation of staff, technology available, and/or exercise programs may become important to communicate.

If the target consumer is presumed ready to select an alternative regimen or facility, minimizing his or her fear in making a selection and conveying a superior reputation become important. Strategies appropriate for this stage for the center for heart diseases would consist of communicating the advantages of treating heart problems and the advantages of choosing the center over competitors.

Finally, at the implementation stage of the consumer decision process, information that facilitates selection should be disseminated. At this stage, the center for heart diseases focuses on communicating hours of service, how an appointment is made, what information will be needed at the appointment, and so forth.

Each stage offers specific opportunities for using marketing communications. If the stage of the decision process can be identified for the target market, this model is a useful tool for devising marketing communication strategies.

DEVELOPING ACTION PROGRAMS

Once the marketing strategy is developed, the action program or the combination of specific steps or tactics that will accomplish the strategy is detailed. The use of Responsibility and Gantt Charting (see chapter 6 for description of these techniques) is best when developing action programs in order to ensure both efficiency and timeliness.

A general rule for developing action programs is this: remember that "everything about an organization talks." In a clinical setting, this idea is best presented by Alward (1983): "Services, employers, facilities, actions and attitudes communicate something about the nursing division and the hospital organization. When these factors are recognized as sources of marketing promotion, their impact can be realistically assessed."

Topor (1986, p. 8) applies this notion in a similar fashion to an educational setting when he cites, "Everything about an institution talks. Everything communicates. The institution's programs, its administration, faculty, students and alumni "speak" about the institution. Items that may at first seem hardly significant still contribute to the institution's image. . . ."

Application of the rule (cited above) to developing action programs means that the marketer needs to consider all avenues and publics when developing tactics. For example, suppose a nursing school has the short-term marketing objective of developing and promoting a master's of nursing administration program for executive nurses in one year. The marketing strategy consists of developing and promoting the program to meet the unique needs of executive nurses and to portray an elitist image for the program. Tactics for achieving this marketing strategy must not only include the development of the program and brochure but also the following:

- Communicating the availability and description of this program to internal and external publics of the school (e.g., other faculty members, secretaries, university administration, and alumni). Certainly, it would be a positive impact upon the program if a potential applicant telephoned the school and had an informed secretary provide him or her with the information required, in a professional manner. The availability of this program also would be appropriately communicated by faculty at professional meetings.

- Applying the elitist "executive" image throughout the delivery of the program (i.e., in the approach of the faculty member, requirements of the courses, communication, policies and procedures regarding the program, etc.). If a faculty member came dressed "for success" to teach class or the executive nurse student were given independence regarding assignment completion, this would be congruent with the "elitist, executive" image.

Suppose in a clinical setting a marketing objective of the nursing department is to develop a reputation of being a professional nursing staff. This theme cannot only be communicated; it also needs to be practiced by the nursing staff. That is, it is not good enough to tell people you are professional—you also need to act it.

While the notion of "everything about an organization talks" is a simplistic one, it is one that needs to be remembered when one is developing action programs, so that avenues for achieving objectives are not overlooked.

IMPLEMENTING THE MARKETING PLAN— HELPFUL HINTS FOR THE COMMUNICATION VARIABLE

Implementation of the product, place, and price variables involve activities that are familiar to nurse administrators; that is, provision of education and nursing care; determination of schedules and locations; and setting the tuition, salary, and/or cost of nursing care. On the other hand, implementing activities to promote nursing products is fairly new to nurse administrators. This section offers techniques useful for implementing activities related to:

- Public service advertising.
- Publicity.
- Advertising.
- Nonconventional promotional techniques.

Public Service Advertising

Public service advertising or donated advertising for obvious reasons is a preferable method of communicating to markets. However, given the greater acceptance of marketing activities by nonprofit organizations, there is increased competition for public service advertising. The first step for someone interested in obtaining public service advertising is to identify what is available. Gaffner (1981) suggests that the best way to identify and obtain public service advertising is to visit each public service director in the local radio and television stations and ask the following questions:

Public Service Announcements (PSAs)

- Does the station offer PSAs and if so, in what time lengths—10, 30, or 60 seconds?
- How often and at what time periods are the PSAs aired during the broadcast day?
- In what format does the station want to receive your information —as a timed written script or as a full news release that station personnel will edit?
- How far in advance does the station want to receive PSA information—one, two, or three weeks?

Public Service Talk Shows

- Does the station have any regularly scheduled guest interview shows?
- If so, are they scheduled daily, weekly, or monthly?
- During what time periods are they scheduled, and on what day of the week?
- What time length are the shows?
- How far in advance does the public service director like to schedule appearances?
- What types are they most interested in airing?

- How often do they want to be advised of potential interviews and in what manner—by a monthly newsletter, phone call, or news release?

Knowledge of this information will enable nurse administrators to exhaust the public service advertising available to them. Public service advertising can be designed to best fit the desires of those who provide this public service. In addition, the meetings or interviews will also cultivate a more personal relationship with the directors of public service advertising, which is advantageous to securing their cooperation.

Publicity

Publicity is also a very attractive method of promotion that is not easily obtained. Publicity is probably even more attractive than public service advertising, given the greater attention span of the audience. Nursing is in a good position for publicity because of the growing interest in the nursing shortage and health care options.

As with public service advertising, it is important, when seeking publicity, that nursing administrators "know their media." Smith (1981) suggests that each newspaper, radio, and television station has its own biases, likes, and dislikes. Knowledge of these peculiarities will increase the ability to secure publicity.

Press releases need to be well written, concise, relevant to current news events, and interesting or attention-getting. Smith (1981) indicates that it is advantageous to back up press releases with personal phone calls and personal letters.

Advertising

Advertising is typically thought of in terms of being done through television, radio, and print (newspapers, journals, brochures) mediums. In the selection of the advertising medium or combination of mediums to be used, the marketing objectives and target markets are considered in light of the characteristics of the medium. Wright, Warner, Winter, and Ziegler (1979) suggest the following characteristics to be considered in selecting advertising mediums:

1. *Selectivity* is the ability of the medium to reach specific target markets. If the objective is to reach the market for a nurse educator's program, a nursing journal is more selective than a radio station. However, during the radio station's "health hour," selectivity is enhanced.

2. *Coverage* is the penetration or size of the audience of a medium in a given area or within a particular market segment. The target market desired impacts the medium's coverage (i.e., while a television advertisement is assumed to have wide coverage, if it is not reaching the desired segment, then the coverage is limited).

3. *Flexibility* is the ease and amount of time required to place an advertisement. In general, newspapers, radio, and direct mail are considered flexible mediums, while television and journals are considered unflexible.

4. *Cost* should be considered in terms of actual dollar amount and in terms of results per dollar spent. If public service advertising is not secured, the cost factor will eliminate the use of television as a medium for most nursing organizations. However, before that decision is made, the administrator ought to consider the cost of the television ads in light of the benefits that may result from the ad.

5. *Editorial environment* refers to the reputation or image of the medium. For television and radio, this characteristic should be considered in light of the time the advertisement would appear. As an example, an advertisement during the radio station's "Top 40" program has a different environment than during a syndicated talk show.

6. *Production quality* is the quality of the medium's appearance. A journal would have a higher production quality than a newspaper.

7. *Permanence* is the length of time an advertisement is displayed. Newspaper advertisements have a longer permanence than radio advertisements. If a lengthy message is to be conveyed, permanence becomes a key factor.

As might be expected, once the mediums have been chosen, the design of the advertisements also depend upon the marketing objective and the target market for the product. In developing the design of an advertisement, Kotler (1982) suggests that an "AIDA" formula be kept in mind. Therefore, advertising should:

A get *A*ttention
I hold *I*nterest
D arouse *D*esire
A obtain *A*ction

Keeping this formula or these criteria in mind when one is designing advertising can be useful for ensuring effectiveness.

Barton and Treadwell (1978) offer the following list of commonly made mistakes in educational advertising, which also applies to most clinical settings:

1. Trying to say too much in too little space (or too little time).
2. Writing copy that interests the institution instead of what interests the target market.
3. Using any available photographs instead of choosing photographs that illustrate the message desired.
4. Trying to communicate the impression that the institution is all things to all people instead of a specialized place for special people.

In addition to trying to avoid these common mistakes, the nursing administrator should also realize the strength of continuity in advertising. Repetition of the same message theme or slogan is a proven method to increase recall and attention-getting power of advertising.

Advertising costs are important for most nursing organizations. Gaffner (1981) offers the following ways to reduce cost when advertising:

1. Do your own production if you have the capabilities and facilities.
2. Develop commercials in a way that the television audio tracks double as radio commercials (this also allows for strong continuity, since the same message is repeated).
3. Use testimonial commercials—they have been determined to be strong and believable.
4. Maintain the same overall theme.

NONCONVENTIONAL PROMOTIONAL TECHNIQUES

The nursing administrator may find it more effective to decide on less traditional promotional techniques. More specifically, in addition to using public service advertising, publicity, television, radio, or print advertising, the following list provides more innovative approaches to promotion:

- *Billboard advertising* has the advantage of permanence for a fairly low cost.
- *Movie theatre advertising* is inexpensive and has potential for meeting specific target markets (i.e., the audience for a particular type of movie can be identified).
- *Newsletter*: a school of nursing or nursing clinic newsletter is an effective method for communicating services and ideas to specific audiences.

- *Sales promotion*: Buttons, sweatshirts, pens, pencils, and other items with the "slogan" of the school or nursing department are effective in reinforcing a theme.
- *Open houses*: A social event is a good method of communicating in educational or clinical settings.
- *Posters* are usually acceptable in nursing clinical and educational settings as well as other target locations.
- *Videos* are a rapidly growing form of promotion that are especially useful when much information is sought by the consumer.
- *Presentations at meetings*: While nurse administrators have recruited students at high schools and nurses at job fairs for some time, also important is the idea of promoting nursing products through presentations at associations, clubs, and other types of group meetings.

EVALUATING THE MARKETING PLAN

Evaluation of the effectiveness of the marketing plan completes the strategic marketing process cycle and provides input to future marketing efforts. As stated earlier, the evaluation of the marketing plan is virtually built-in through the specification of detailed objectives and time frames.

Evaluation research of marketing programs attempts to measure results that can be attributed to the marketing strategy. Comparing results over time and having baseline data become important when one evaluates marketing effectiveness (Smith, 1982). The design of the marketing analysis includes information needs that address marketing effectiveness.

Following are some other examples of ways to evaluate marketing effectiveness:

- For different promotional techniques, use different addresses or telephone numbers. The number of inquiries drawn from the different mediums can be determined.
- As part of record-keeping practices such as applications and admitting forms, ask questions regarding marketing strategies (e.g., have you heard our slogan on TV or radio?).
- As part of evaluation surveys, ask questions related to marketing effectiveness.

Results from the evaluation of the marketing plan become an input to the marketing analysis stage, and the strategic marketing process begins once again.

SUMMARY

The strategic marketing process, like any administrative practice, is far simpler to conceptualize than operationalize within an organization. It is for this reason that this chapter focused on providing practical techniques and strategies for implementing the strategic marketing process.

First and foremost, the marketing effort needs to be marketed to the various publics of the organization. This chapter advocated the need to organize the marketing analysis into organizational, competitive, and market phases, and it provided examples of possible designs of the phases. The importance and techniques for exhausting secondary data sources and conducting efficient primary data collection methods were explained and illustrated.

Strategies for determining marketing opportunities and threats, as well as segmenting markets, were detailed. The chapter provided techniques for developing marketing strategies, including considering the five patterns of coverage available; determining competitor's position and the marketing mix; examining the stage of the product life cycle; and employing a consumer decision model.

The importance of developing explicit objectives, goals, and detailed action plans was emphasized. Finally, helpful hints for operationalizing the communication variable and evaluating marketing programs were provided.

REFERENCES

Alward, R. R. (1983). A marketing approach to nursing administration (Part II). *Journal of Nursing Administration, 13*(4), 18–22.

Armstrong, D. M., Amo, E., Duer, A. L., Hanson, M., Hijeck, T., Kaworski, P., & Young, S. (1985). Marketing opportunities for a nursing department in a changing economic environment. *Nursing Administration Quarterly, 10*(1), 1–10.

Barton, D. W., & Treadwell, D. R. (1978). Marketing: A synthesis of institutional soul-searching and aggressiveness. *New Directions for Higher Education, 21*, 77–84.

Clifford, D. K. (1980). Managing the product life cycle. In P. Kotler and K. Cox (Eds.), *Marketing management and strategy* (pp. 175–181). Englewood Cliffs, NJ: Prentice Hall.

Gaffner, R. H. (1981). Marketing and the electronic media. In W. Keim and M. Keim (Eds.), *New directions for community colleges: Marketing the program* ([36] pp. 45–53). San Francisco: Jossey-Bass.

Gaither, G. H. (1980). Some tools and techniques of market research for students. In R. E. Murphy and E. R. Laczinak (Eds.), *Marketing education: Current status and a view for the 1980s* (pp. 31–67). Chicago: American Marketing Association.

Gollattscheck, J. F. (1981). Caution! Marketing may be hazardous to your institutional health. In W. Keim and M. Keim (Eds.), *New directions for community colleges: Marketing the program* ([36], pp. 99–105). San Francisco: Jossey-Bass.

Kotler, P. (1982). *Marketing for nonprofit organizations* (2nd ed.). Englewood Cliffs, NJ: Prentice-Hall.

Larkin, P. G. (1980). Market research methods for improving college responsiveness. In R. E. Murphy and E. R. Laczinak (Eds.), *Marketing education: Current status and a view for the 1980s* (pp. 11–30). Chicago: American Marketing Association.

MacStravic, R. E. S. (1985). *Managing health care marketing communications*. Rockville, MD: Aspen Systems.

Smith, B. A. W. (1981). Marketing and the printed media: Getting the promotional job done. In W. Keim and M. Keim (Eds.), *New directions for community colleges: Marketing the program* ([36] pp. 39–44). San Francisco: Jossey-Bass.

Smith, R. M. (1982). Knowledge is power. *Case Currents, 14,* 8–12.

Topor, R. (1983). *Marketing higher education: A practical guide*. Washington, DC: Council for Advancement and Support of Education.

Wright, J. S., Warner, D. S., Winter, W. L., & Zeigler, S. K. (1977). *Advertising* (4th ed.). New York: McGraw-Hill.

5

Program Evaluation

Carolyn Feher Waltz

The imperative is clear: Nurses must be accountable not only for quality care, but also for providing important audiences with evidence that nursing *does* make a difference. A well-executed, comprehensive program evaluation is the key to success in meeting this need. Writing on the need for reform in program evaluation, Cronbach et al. (1980) identify the standard for judging an evaluation as its contribution to public thinking and the quality of service provided subsequent to the evaluation. They further assert:

> An evaluation pays off to the extent that it offers ideas pertinent to pending actions and people think more clearly as a result. To enlighten, it must do more than amass good data, . . . timely evaluation should distribute information to the persons rightfully concerned, and those hearers should take the information into their thinking . . . broadly speaking an evaluation ought to inform and improve the operations of the social system. (pp. 63–64)

This emerging view of evaluation and its potential for impact extends far beyond prior expectations of the outcome of evaluation. It places new emphasis on the importance of carrying out well-designed and well-executed program evaluations in nursing that are sensitive to the decision-making needs of a wide audience.

PURPOSES FOR EVALUATION

Evaluation is a decision-making process that leads to suggestions for action to maintain and/or improve the effectiveness and efficiency of programs and participants. It is a primary mechanism for assessing the effects of strategic planning and marketing, as well as for conveying the importance of nursing. A comprehensive, ongoing program evaluation in nursing can serve many useful purposes, including:

1. Clarification and definition of program goals and objectives.
2. Clarification and definition of the goals and objectives of those who participate in the program.
3. Improvement in the care provided to clients.
4. Improvement in program inputs, operations, and outcomes.
5. Determination of progress toward the achievement of program and participant goals and objectives.
6. Maintenance of strengths and elimination of weaknesses on the part of participants.
7. Maintenance of program strengths and elimination of program weaknesses.
8. Motivation of participants in the program.
9. Provision of psychological security for participants and clients that is likely to result in increased client and participant satisfaction, reduction in burnout, turnover, attrition, etc.
10. Development of more relevant, reliable, and valid means for communicating the results of nursing efforts to others.
11. Determination of the overall program value (e.g., cost efficiency, cost/benefit of the nursing program for participants, administrators, and clients immediately and over longer periods of time).
12. Establishment, maintenance, and/or improvement of standards to meet legal and/or professional credentialing (Staropoli & Waltz, 1978, pp. 84–87).

PROGRAM EVALUATION PRINCIPLES AND PRACTICES

The principles that govern evaluation in nursing are the same as those that apply to the evaluation of any programmatic endeavor. Whenever an evaluation is undertaken, one needs to consider the following:

WHO is to be involved
WHY the evaluation is being conducted
WHAT is to be the subject of the evaluation
HOW the evaluation is to proceed
WHEN evaluation is to occur

The unique character of nursing impacts when strategies and techniques to implement these principles are designed and/or selected. Then, differences between evaluating programs in nursing and in other fields emerge.

Ideally, whenever a program evaluation is undertaken, the principles described below should be taken into account.

WHO

1. The individual(s) responsible and accountable for conducting the evaluation should be identified early and explicitly.
2. Evaluation is most relevant when it builds on and involves the audience for its results.
3. If evaluation is to accomplish its purposes, then those who plan and implement the evaluation should be involved in decision making as well.

WHY

The general aims of evaluation are to:

1. Determine the extent to which program goals and objectives are met.
2. Provide answers to questions that arise from a number of sources and perspectives.

WHAT

1. Goals and objectives that reflect the outcomes expected as a result of the program experience.
2. Specific questions and/or concerns identified by the audience for program results; that is, those who will make decisions about the program.

HOW

1. A procedure for how decisions will be made on the basis of evalua tion results must be established and agreed upon before data is collected.
2. In determining the types of information to be collected, it is necessary to plan for the collection of information that the various audiences will be willing to use for decision making.
3. Progress in meeting program goals and objectives must be measured in terms of observable behaviors.
4. Methods employed for the collection of data should be specific to purpose, varied in type, multiple in number, and should have the characteristics deemed essential to a "good" tool:
   a. reliability
   b. validity
   c. specificity
   d. practical design
   e. utility in diagnosing strengths and weaknesses
   f. inclusion of only factors crucial to making decisions

WHEN

Evaluation should be an ongoing activity that begins at first identification of the need for a program, proceeds throughout the planning and implementing phases, and continues after expiration of the program:

1. Within any program, evaluation should occur frequently in order to construct an accurate picture of progress.
2. Evaluation should not be attempted until after participants have had an opportunity to be involved in the program.
3. Evaluative efforts should reflect a progression in outcomes from simple to complex and from one stage of implementation to the next.
4. When evaluation serves as a mechanism for ongoing improvement of the program, it should occur before, during, and after the program at regular times designated for the purpose.
5. To assess the attainment of objectives, evaluation should occur prior to the program, during the program, immediately upon completion, and at later intervals.

Evaluation should occur at those points in time at which decision-makers will be willing to take action, that is, to make changes, if necessary, on the basis of results (Staropoli & Waltz, 1978, pp. 84–88).

Standards for the practice of evaluation are available from two sources: (1) *Standards for Evaluation of Educational Programs, Projects, and Materials* (1981), which describes 30 standards to be used both to guide the conduct of evaluation of programs, projects, and materials, and also to judge the soundness of such evaluations (Stufflebeam & Madaus, 1983); and (2) *Toward Reform of Program Evaluation* (Cronbach, 1980), in which Cronbach et al. argue the need for a comprehensive transformation of evaluation. Taking their lead from Martin Luther, they present their arguments and recommendations as 95 theses. An abbreviated summary of these theses is also available in *Evaluation Models*, edited by Madaus, Scriven, and Stufflebeam (1983).

PROGRAM EVALUATION IN NURSING

Differences between evaluating programs in nursing and in other fields emerge when these evaluation principles are operationalized. When a framework for evaluation is selected, the unique and specific characteristics of nursing and its settings must be taken into consideration. Similarly, the strategies and techniques for evaluation implementation must be tailored to the particular nursing program and setting.

In nursing, when responsibility for the evaluation is determined, too often the services of an external evaluator are sought. Perhaps this results in part from the prevailing misconception that evaluation can only be objective when conducted by an outsider and/or from feelings of inadequacy. External evaluators are expensive, with limited time to give to the evaluation. As a result, the outside evaluator generally completes the task when the evaluation has been designed and implemented, and decisionmakers are then left with results they too often find irrelevant and/or difficult to understand—and virtually impossible to act upon.

Evaluation is a stated function of essentially every nurse's job description whether the nurse is a practitioner, educator, or administrator. If the involvement of external evaluators is limited to a minimum and individuals and groups within the organization are held accountable for the evaluation responsibilities and functions that are part of their jobs, not only can evaluation cost be reduced considerably, but also evaluation easily becomes an ongoing aspect of the day-to-day operation. The ultimate purpose for evaluation (i.e., decisionmaking) is apt to occur more efficiently, since the designers and implementors re-main accountable. This approach to evaluation is likely to be most suc-cessful when a master plan is first designed to integrate evaluation ac-tivities required to evaluate the program, so that an individual or group can in fact implement the aspects of the evaluation inherent in their job without the added burden of being thoroughly familiar with the whole. This approach to evaluation is evident in many agencies where internal evaluators, such as directors of research and evaluation or quality assurance, coordinate the evaluation effort.

In nursing settings, the success of any evaluation rests solely on its ability to generate information that will be useful in decisionmaking. Therefore, a more comprehensive approach to evaluation will allow for a greater flexibility in making judgments at all levels of an organiza-tion. In this respect, it is not sufficient to focus evaluation only on the extent to which goals and objects are met; attention also must be paid to questions and concerns of individuals inside and outside the organi-zation, people who make decisions about a program. Ideally, evaluation in nursing should consider inputs, processes, outcomes, and the inter-relationships among the three, as well as their interaction with their environment, but to address evaluation in this manner can be costly. Therefore, cost is a factor in determining focus for a given evaluation.

In general, then, the best evaluation is one that focuses on the behav-ior critical to achieving goals and objectives, and upon information needed for decisionmaking. It is inefficient to attempt to assess every-thing in regard to a single objective and/or evaluation question; only factors crucial to making judgments should be considered. Those in-volved in each aspect of the evaluation should be identified during the planning stages with the idea kept in mind that different decisionmak-ers may need similar information in different forms. By identifying decisionmakers during the design of the evaluation, it becomes possible to:

1. Economize by using one method to obtain the information needed by several different audiences, thereby eliminating the need to gather information in one form and then subsequently gather the same information in a different form.

2. Avoid costly redundancies in effort.

3. Identify critical questions, as well as those that might be eliminated from the evaluation, by prioritizing evaluation efforts on the basis of the relative number and importance of the decisionmakers in need of a particular type of evaluative information.

4. Involve various decisionmakers in the determination of the type of information they deem acceptable as a basis for decisionmaking, hence increasing the specificity of the evaluation effort as well as decreasing the potential for information to be deemed irrelevant at decision-making time.

5. Gain the cooperation of decisionmakers in the establishment of rules for how judgments will be made on the basis of results prior to the data collection, so that when information is collected, the right information can be routed to the appropriate audiences in a timely, relevant, and least-costly manner (Waltz & Bond, 1985, p. 260).

It is imperative that effective exchange of evaluation information occur and that evaluation timetables and procedures be communicated and understood at all levels of the organization. When dates for the completion of various evaluation activities are defined, effectively communicated, and adhered to, availability of data for decisionmaking is apt to be more timely (Waltz & Bond, 1985, p. 260).

Thus, in the selection of an approach for evaluating programs in nursing, a framework selected must provide for:

1. Decisionmaking, especially as it relates to program and participant effectiveness and efficiency.

2. The information needs of various audiences or decisionmakers inside and outside the organization.

3. Evaluation of all aspects of the program, including inputs, processes, outcomes, their interrelationships with each other, and the environment in which they occur.

4. Conduct of the evaluation by an internal evaluator.

5. Utilization of a variety of different evaluation methods to implement a variety of different evaluation activities.

6. Collection of evaluation data before, during, immediately after the program, and later.

7. Efficiency and cost containment as it relates to the conduct of the evaluation.

Evaluation Prototypes

As noted previously, one needs to take into account the nature of nursing and nursing programs and to select an approach that provides for the conditions listed in the preceding section. The viewpoints presented here are those of leading authors whose works have served as prototypes for the large number of specific evaluation approaches appearing in the literature. Each model characterizes its author's view of the main concepts involved in evaluation and provides guidelines for using these concepts to arrive at defensible descriptions, judgments, and recommendations. These views correspond to what Stufflebeam and Webster (1983) characterize as idealized or "model" views of how to sort out and address the problems encountered in conducting evaluations. They include: Tyler's Objective-Based Evaluation, Accreditation/Certification Evaluation, Stake's Client-Centered Evaluation, Stufflebeam's Decision-Oriented Evaluation, Taba's Experimental-Research Evaluation, and Scriven's Consumer-Oriented Evaluation. Also discussed is Utilization-Focused Evaluation as conceived by Patton.

Objective-Based Evaluation (Tyler)

Tyler, often referred to as the father of educational evaluation, is generally acknowledged to be the pioneer in objective-based evaluation. Others who developed variations of his objective-based evaluation model include Blood, Englehart, Furst, Hill, and Krathwohl (1956), Metfessel and Michael (1967), Popham (1969), Provus (1971), and Hammond (1972). This model has been the most prevalent type used in educational evaluation (Stufflebeam & Webster, 1983).

The key emphasis in Tyler's model (Tyler, 1942, 1949; Stufflebeam & Webster, 1983) is objectives—specifically, because the model was developed for educational programs, instructional objectives. In this view, the purpose of evaluation is to determine the extent to which prespecified, behaviorally stated objectives are achieved by learners, before, during, and after an educational experience, that is, immediately following the program and one to five years later. The crux of the evaluation activities is the careful formulation of educational objectives stated in terms of student behavior. These objectives are derived from an analysis of student and societal needs, content, educational philosophy, and learning theories. The primary viewpoint used to delimit the objectives and, therefore, what will be studied, is the curriculum, supervisor, and teacher. Outside experts are involved in two ways: (1) specifying objectives, especially as they reflect societal needs; and (2) measurement.

Tyler recognizes the need for a variety of evaluation devices to assess cognitive and affective domains, and he advocates more than paper and pencil measures. In selecting evaluation measures, he stresses reliability, validity, and objectivity. Multiple-data sources and tools are used to determine whether or not objectives are being met, identify strengths and weaknesses in the curriculum, and promote decisions regarding program alteration. Faculty members play an important role in this approach as those who conceptualize objectives and administer evaluation tools.

The major strengths of the framework stem from its emphasis on the need for clear specification of behavioral objectives for assessing learner outcomes and the fact that it provides for a check on the degree of congruence between objectives and the learning experiences provided for students. The approach has been criticized for not providing for examination of the quality of goals and procedures for measuring goal attainment (Scriven, 1967). It has also been criticized for being focused on outputs, having a means–end orientation, and for ignoring processes (Popham, 1975; Werner, 1978; Saylor & Alexander, 1974). In Scriven's terms, it is largely summative. Stake (1976) has also expressed concern that it is not process oriented because of its lack of concern with describing phenomena encountered as a program progresses. Stufflebeam and Webster (1983) note that such studies lead to information that is of little use in program improvement and far too narrow in scope to constitute a sound basis for judging the worth of a program.

While the model has some utility for evaluating nursing programs, especially educational programs, it does not provide a number of essential conditions. A positive aspect of the approach from the nursing perspective is its focus on behaviorally stated cognitive and affective objectives and their measurement, especially the need for employing multiple methods in assessing outcomes immediately upon completion of the program and later. This is an important consideration in a practice-oriented profession such as nursing. However, performance objectives, which are especially important in nursing programs, are not emphasized, limiting their utility for nursing. In nursing, it is essential that attention be given within the context of program evaluation to the quality of goals and that the focus of objective evaluation extend beyond student-centered objectives to include, as well, objectives that center on faculty, clients, curriculum, organizational structure, and environment.

The framework's utility in nursing is diminished by its reliance on an external evaluator and its narrow definition of the audience as educational administrators and faculty. The major audiences for the results of nursing evaluations are far more inclusive than are provided for;

they include, but are not limited to, funding agencies, consumers of services, accrediting groups, prospective faculty, and students.

Outcomes are a major concern in nursing and warrant more attention than they receive. However, a focus on outcomes to the exclusion of other important program components is neither feasible nor useful. If evaluations are to generate information useful for decisionmaking by the variety of audiences, they must provide for the collection of data regarding inputs, processes, the environment, and their interrelationships, as well as outcomes. Similarly, performance as well as cognition and affect must be a focus of the evaluation. Attention to the use of reliable, valid, and objective measurements is a plus.

Accreditation/Certification Evaluation

Accreditation in education was pioneered by the College Entrance Examination Board around 1901. Since then, the accreditation function has been implemented and expanded by associations of secondary schools, and colleges along with their associated regional accrediting agencies across the United States, and by many other accrediting and certifying bodies. The purpose of accreditation/certification is to determine whether institutions, programs, or personnel should be approved to perform specified functions. This determination is usually made on the basis of self-study and self-reporting by the individual and/or institution, using guidelines that have been adopted by the accrediting or certifying body (Floden, 1983; Stufflebeam & Webster, 1983).

This approach is best exemplified by the National League for Nursing (NLN) accreditation process. The purpose is to review content and procedures for instruction. For example, the two stated purposes for NLN accreditation are to (1) assist the school by serving as a guide to faculty developing and improving educational programs and as a framework for self-evaluation, and (2) assist NLN in the appraisal of an educational program in terms of philosophy and purposes of the school. Methods include a self-study by faculty followed by judgment by professional peers regarding the quality of the program. Primary data collection, interpretation, and recommendations are initiated by program faculty and administrators. The program is assessed regarding relative strengths and weaknesses using criteria developed by member agencies of the accrediting group. Focuses for evaluation usually include organization and administration of the educational program, policies regarding students and faculty, the curriculum, resources, facilities, and services. Following the self-study, the school is visited by a team of peer observers who verify, clarify, amplify, and validate the evidence presented in the self-study report. The report of the visit, along with the self-study, are then submitted to a board of review, where formal judgments regarding the program are made. The key viewpoints reflected in the evaluation are those of faculty and administrators of the program, with outside experts not included unless authentication by outside peers is warranted.

The main advantage of the accreditation/certification evaluation is that it aids lay persons in making informal judgments about the quality of institutions and the qualifications of personnel (Stufflebeam & Webster, 1983) and that it stresses internal responsibility for evaluation. The approach has been characterized as very subjective, largely because it ignores the views of people outside the organization/accrediting agency. Another difficulty with the approach stems from the fact that guidelines of accrediting and certifying bodies typically emphasize process, not outcome criteria. Stufflebeam and Webster (1983, p. 32) also note that the self-study and visitation processes offer many opportunities for corruption and inept performance.

This approach is extensively used in nursing. It makes administrators and faculty accountable for the evaluation activities inherent in their job functions and responsibilities. Unfortunately, its overall utility as the sole approach to evaluating the total program is limited by its emphasis on processes, subjectivity, and internal judgments. To be used successfully and comprehensively, this emphasis would need to be balanced by equal attention to more objective methods, greater involvement on the part of outsiders to reduce biases, and expansion of the utility of results for a larger number of decisionmakers. The approach does not give sufficient attention to the effects of the educational program or to extrinsic, objective criteria for evaluation of its products. In a practice-oriented profession such as nursing, outcomes cannot be assessed adequately without involving the consumers of services.

Client-Centered Evaluation (Stake)

Stake is the forerunner of client-centered evaluations. This approach takes the local autonomy view where people who are involved in a program evaluate it, then use the evaluation to improve it. The purpose of such an evaluation is to help people in a local setting to understand the operations of their program, the ways the operations are valued by the people affected by them, and the ways they are valued by people who are expert in the program area (Stufflebeam & Webster, 1983).

Stake's Countenance Model (Green & Lewis, 1986; House, 1980; Patton, 1980; Stake, 1967, 1976, 1983) is used frequently in evaluating programs in both nursing education and service. In this approach, description and judgment are viewed as the two basic acts of evaluation. Descriptive and judgmental acts are distinguished according to the *antecedent* (conditions that existed prior to the program processes), *transaction* (succession of engagements that comprise the program process), and *outcome* phases of the program (immediate and long-term effects of a program on participants, clients, and others in the community). Both descriptions and judgments must be described fully according to whether they refer to what was intended by those affected by the program and what the evaluator, who is external to the program, actually observes. Stake recognizes the antipathy of many to objectives and, therefore, sees the role of the evaluator to identify behavioral objectives to facilitate data collection, but he does not impose this requirement on those internal to the organization. Those inside the organization may describe intents in any manner they desire, since the major purpose is to report the ways that different people see the program. Methods, largely subjective, typically employed are the case study, adversary reports, sociodrama, and what Stake (1983) has called "responsive evaluation." Evaluation activities are designed to ascertain what the audiences want to know, and to observe and gather opinions. Audiences are defined broadly to include the public, content experts, professional groups, staff, and so forth, and the key viewpoint delimiting the evaluation is that of the audience for the final report.

The major strength of the model rests with its broad view of the program and of conflicting expectations. Another strength, noted by Stufflebeam and Webster (1983), is that it is an action–research approach in which people implementing programs are helped to conduct their own evaluation. Its main weakness is its lack of external credibility and its susceptibility to bias on the part of people in the local setting, since, in effect, they have great control over the evaluation. In assessing his own model, Stake has recognized the possibility of stirring up value conflicts among people whose opinions are sought and notes that the model does not provide for examining causes, and that the use of description tends to omit the use of objective measuring devices.

Stake's approach has been used extensively, and it has been developed further by Rippey (1973), McDonald (1975), and Guba (1978). Regarding its utility for nursing, it is perhaps the most complete of the approaches available in terms of its concern with audience needs for information. As noted earlier, it is imperative that evaluation methods used in nursing address the specific concerns of respective audiences, inside and outside the program under assessment. Stake also highlights the importance of judgments, while other existing models do not directly address this important aspect of evaluation, even though, by definition, evaluation is a decision-making process. What limits the model's use in nursing is its overreliance on subjective methods and opinions.

Decision-Oriented Evaluation (Stufflebeam)

This approach to evaluation emanating from the work of Stufflebeam emphasizes that evaluation should be used proactively to help improve a program, as well as retroactively to judge its worth (Stufflebeam & Webster, 1983). Basically, the purpose of such an evaluation is to provide a knowledge and value base for making and defending decisions. Others who have contributed to a decision-oriented concept of evaluation are Alkin (1969), Reinhard (1972), Taylor (1974), Ashburn (1972), Guba (1976), Merriman (1968), Ott (1967), Walker (1974), and Webster (1975).

Stufflebeam's CIPP (context, input, process, and product) *Model* (Green & Lewis, 1986; Patton, 1980; Stufflebeam, 1966, 1967, 1969; Phi Delta Kappa Commission on Evaluation, 1971; Stufflebeam & Webster, 1983) emphasizes decisionmaking. In this approach, evaluation is viewed as a process of delineating, obtaining, and providing useful information for judging decision alternatives. The primary purpose of evaluation is to facilitate rational and continuing decisionmaking. In the CIPP model, evaluators and decisionmakers are distinct, a fact too often overlooked by those in nursing who employ the approach with an internal evaluator. In this view, the evaluator collects and presents information needed by decisionmakers to assess the worth of the program. Stufflebeam strongly advocates that the evaluator be external to the program to ensure objectivity in the evaluation effort.

Context evaluation has as its specific purpose the determination of objectives by isolating problems and unmet needs in the setting. Context evaluation provides the rationale for the selection of specific program objectives and establishes the boundaries of the system to be evaluated leading to *planning decisions.*

Input evaluation provides information for deciding how to utilize resources and what resources to employ in meeting program goals. The end product of this type of evaluation is an assessment of one or more procedural techniques in terms of cost-benefit analysis leading to *structural decisions.*

Process evaluation provides periodic feedback to designers and those responsible for implementation after a specific program has been approved and instituted. Its purpose is to identify any deficiencies between program conception and implementation. Decisions following process evaluation are referred to as *implementation decisions*.

Product evaluation measures and interprets achievement resulting from the program and determines the extent to which program objectives are met. Measures of outcomes are obtained at the end of the program and as often as necessary to determine whether to continue, terminate, or modify the program and, therefore, lead to what Stufflebeam refers to as *recycling decisions*.

A main advantage of decision-oriented evaluation is that it encourages the continuous and systematic use of evaluation in efforts to plan and implement programs that meet needs. It also presents a rationale for accountable decisions made in the course of implementing a program (Stufflebeam & Webster, 1983). The primary audiences in this view are program directors and administrators; thus, the audience is somewhat limited in definition, and there is a danger that efficiency may be overvalued and organizational aims undervalued.

Unfortunately, the model's utility in nursing is limited by the fact that evaluators and decisionmakers are viewed as separate and distinct entities. In nursing, not only is internal evaluation more economically feasible, but there is also a long history of utilizing experts without involvement of those who make decisions resulting in a lack of action on the basis of evaluation results. This is often the case because evaluation is limited in scope, information collected is not readily useful for making decisions, or more often is irrelevant to the needs of decisionmakers. Also, the audience for results in nursing is broader and more inclusive than program administrators. Within nursing settings, many types of decisions need to be made at many different levels by different individuals within the organization. Also, there are a number of external audiences of import, including a host of consumer-oriented decisions to be made. As noted earlier, evaluation traditionally has been part of the functions and responsibilities of nurses in all settings; it is not something that should be given over to external evaluators.

The CIPP model is attentive to inputs, processes, outcomes, and the context in which they occur, as well as to cost benefit, a component not explicitly addressed by most other models. The process focus on discrepancies may lead to a tendency to look for problems or weaknesses as a result of the evaluation effort. In the evaluation of nursing programs, it is imperative that equal importance be given to identifying program strengths and what works, so as to maintain the quality of programs as well as improve them. Other aspects of the model useful in nursing include the recognition of the need for immediate and long-range assessment of outcomes and recycling decisions, and the inclusion of both formative and summative evaluation methods.

Experimental-Research Evaluation (Taba)

The experimental-research evaluation was pioneered by Taba (1962, 1966), Campbell and Stanley (1963), Cronbach and Snow (1969), and Lindquist (1953). Others who have developed the methodology substantially for evaluation use are Glass and Maguire (1968), Suchman (1967), and Wiley and Bock (1967). The usual purpose of the experimental-research evaluation is to determine causal relationships between specified independent and dependent variables.

In Taba's Social Studies Model, an experimental-research design approach is utilized to determine cause-and-effect relationships. The major purpose for evaluating is to determine the effectiveness of specific program plans and approaches to program development. Thus, the central function of the evaluation is validation of hypotheses upon which the program is based. Another important function of the evaluation, according to Taba, is to provide information regarding the quality of the program by assessing strengths and weaknesses in outcomes, exercising experimental control, and systematic variation. The approach involves four major steps. First, it is necessary to decide what kinds of evaluation data are needed in relation to objectives, factors affecting program processes, and methods. Second, it is necessary to select and develop instruments and procedures for evaluating. Third, information is analyzed to develop hypotheses regarding possible changes in the program. Fourth, it is necessary to transfer hypotheses into action. The major viewpoints directing evaluation in this scheme are those of the researcher and theorists.

Typical methods used are experimental and quasiexperimental designs. It is notable that the sources of questions investigated in the evaluation are those of researchers and program developers and not usually the constituency, practitioners, or financial sponsors (Stufflebeam & Webster, 1983). The main advantage of the approach is that it provides strong methods for establishing evidence of causal relationships between process and outcome variables. Problems, however, stem from the fact that the strategy is generally not workable in field settings and provides a much narrower range of information than is needed to evaluate programs. In addition, such evaluations tend to provide terminal information that is not too useful for guiding the program development process (Stufflebeam & Webster, 1983).

In regard to the approach's utility in nursing, it is necessary to note that the employment of an experimental-research design precludes the ongoing utilization of feedback to make necessary improvements in the program as it is implemented because of the necessity for tight control of the experimental situation and a rigid design. In situations in which this approach is used alone for the evaluation, a dilemma soon arises. That is, when the need for modification in the program implementation becomes evident, one has two choices for action. Either the needed changes can be ignored and the evaluation preserved at the expense of program quality and integrity, or the necessary changes can be made, thus nullifying the evaluation effort. For this reason, experimental research evaluation is best employed in nursing in combination with other, less rigorous methods that allow for responsiveness to the program needs, when necessary. This approach has its greatest utility in nursing when descriptive methods have been employed and subsequent, more rigorous follow-up is required to provide additional answers to more specific evaluation questions. It also has its greatest use in situations where it is possible to randomly assign subjects to treatments, a control group is needed and available, and cause-and-effect relationships are of prime interest. It should be kept in mind, however, that this is but one of many types of studies and that a comprehensive evaluation of a nursing program ought to allow for the conduct of different studies employing a variety of methods. The major criteria for selecting a specific design for evaluating in nursing should be the usefulness of the analysis for reaching rational decisions. Reasons for using nonexperimental designs in nursing evaluation are as follows: (1) most nursing program evaluations are aimed toward defining, describing, and determining effects of conditions as they exist or have been developed by planners; (2) nurses frequently become evaluators and lack the knowledge and experience in research design and statistics; and (3) limited resources in terms of time, money, and consultation services are available to most nursing programs. Another major limitation of this approach for nursing is that it ignores processes per se.

Consumer-Oriented Evaluation (Scriven)

Scriven (1983) pioneered the consumer-oriented evaluation, in which the evaluator is the "enlightened surrogate conscience" (Stufflebeam &

Webster, 1983). Glass (1969) has been an avid supporter and further developer of Scriven's work. The purpose of such an approach is to judge the relative merits of alternative program goods and services and, thereby, to help taxpayers and practitioners to make wise choices in spending (Stufflebeam & Webster, 1983). Questions for study within the context of such an approach are derived from society, constituents of institutions, and—especially—from the evaluator's frame of reference. Methods include checklists, needs assessments, goal-free evaluation, experimental and quasiexperimental designs, modus operandi analysis, and cost analysis (Scriven, 1974; Green & Lewis, 1986; Patton, 1980; Worthen & Sanders, 1973).

Scriven (1967) coined the terms *formative* and *summative evaluation*. Formative evaluation is used during program development as a means of identifying strengths and weaknesses and making adjustments in content and methods. This type of evaluation contributes to improvement of a program in its development phase by providing continuous feedback regarding strengths and weaknesses. Summative evaluation is used to assess the terminal outcomes of a program and focuses on collection and examination of data after program completion to determine the extent to which the program has achieved intended goals. In Scriven's view, the goal of evaluation is judging the merit or worth of a program. According to him, evaluation is a methodological activity that consists simply in the gathering and combining of performance criteria with a weighted set of goal scales to yield either comparative or numerical ratings and in the justification of (a) the data-gathering instruments, (b) the weighing, and (c) the selection of criteria. In explaining this definition, he asserts that evaluation should not only provide information regarding instruments but also should arrive at and report judgments. Instruments, in this sense, are described broadly to include programs, procedures, processes, personnel, and equipment.

Scriven further distinguishes between *intrinsic* and *pay-off evaluation*. Intrinsic evaluation involves assessment of such diverse phenomena as content, goals, procedures, and activities, while payoff evaluation examines the effects of these phenomena on participants in the program. *Goal-free evaluation* (Scriven, 1972) is a means for determining the actual effects, not just the intended effects, of a program. In this view, the evaluator gathers data based on the actual effects of the program and assesses their impact on meeting program needs, without knowing what goals had been specified.

A main advantage of consumer-oriented evaluation is that is has high credibility with consumer groups (Stufflebeam & Webster, 1983). The main disadvantage is that it is so independent from practitioners that it may not assist them to do a better job of serving consumers. Also, the approach requires a highly credible and competent expert plus sufficient resources to allow the expert to conduct a thorough study. Often this approach is too costly to be carried out well and produces faulty, unrealistic data (Stufflebeam & Webster, 1983). The utility of goal-free evaluation is limited in nursing by its emphasis on inputs and outputs, to the exclusion of processes, its reliance on an external evaluator, its limited audience, and high cost to conduct.

Utilization-Focused Evaluation (Patton)

Rutman (1980), in discussing the practice of evaluation, notes that a successful evaluation (one that results in usable findings) is most apt to result when the evaluation (1) focuses on effectiveness, (2) examines operating programs, (3) relies on scientific methods, (4) pays attention to process and outcome, (5) measures goals and effects, and (6) meets information needs of decisionmakers. He contends that cutting across the evaluation-model options are a full range of methods possibilities, the choice in any particular evaluation to be determined by the purpose for the evaluation, and the nature of the evaluation process.

The utilization-focused approach to evaluation (Patton, 1980; Rutman, 1980) represents an attempt to move beyond models to the practice of evaluation. This view presents an evaluation process for making decisions about the content of an evaluation, but the content itself is not specified or implied in advance. Thus, any of the models discussed here, or adaptations and combinations of these models, might emerge as the guiding direction in utilization-focused work. In addition, utilization-focused evaluation is not a model but rather a strategy for making evaluation decisions (Patton, 1980).

Patton's utilization-focused evaluation represents a flexible approach to the selection of evaluation methods in which qualitative methods are highlighted as appropriate, useful, and legitimate for certain evaluation situations. However, he does not preclude the use of quantitative methods within the approach but, rather, he sees a variety of paradigms as appropriate and useful. In this view, the evaluator is "active-reactive-adaptive" in working with decisionmakers and information users to focus evaluation questions and make methods decisions. In essence, the evaluator is a negotiator who strives to obtain the best possible design and the most useful answers to evaluation questions within the real world of politics, people, and methodological prejudice (Patton, 1980, p. 18). The approach begins with the identification and organization of specific, relevant decisionmakers and information users who will employ the information that the evaluation produces. The evaluator works with these people, often organized as a task force, to focus relevant evaluation questions. From these questions flow the appropriate research methods and data analysis techniques. Plans for utilization of findings are made prior to data collection. Program outcomes are evaluated in light of program processes (referred to by Patton as implementors) to provide direction for action, that is, to obtain information regarding what produces observable outcomes and to understand how programs and why programs deviate from intended plans and expectations (Patton, 1980, p. 84).

In order to function in this manner, the evaluator must have a large repertoire of methods and techniques available to use on a variety of problems. The evaluator works directly with decisionmakers to design an evaluation that includes any and all data that will help shed light on evaluation questions, given the constraints of resources and time. Emphasis is placed on research designs that are relevant, rigorous, understandable, and able to produce results that are reliable, valid, and believable. A variety of data collection techniques and design approaches are used, as are multiple methods and triangulation of observations.

The major strengths of this view stem from its concern with the utilization of results in making decisions and its broad view of the appropriateness of varied paradigms and methods in different situations within the context of a given evaluation. Patton refers to this as an approach that replaces competition between different paradigms for research with a "paradigm of choices" (1980, p. 20). Disadvantages result from the cost to employ such diverse and varied paradigms and methods, political considerations that may come into play as a result of the relationship between evaluator and decisionmakers, and the narrowness of training in methods available to most evaluators.

The ideas in this view regarding the use of alternative methods and paradigms have certain applicability in nursing, as does the notion of utilization of results in the real world. The disadvantages noted above limit to some extent the approach's usefulness in nursing.

Table 1 presents a summary of the WHO, WHY, WHAT, WHEN, HOW, and AUDIENCES addressed by the models for evaluation that have served as prototypes for program evaluation in a variety of different fields and settings. It is evident that while all of the prototypes discussed contribute in some manner to the conditions necessary for

Table 1
Prototypes for Program Evaluation

Model/Prototype	Who	Why	What	When	How	Major Audiences
Tyler's Objective-based Evaluation	External evaluator	Measure student progress toward objectives	Inputs/outputs, student-centered behavioral objectives	Before, during immediately after, 1–5 years later	Specific cognitive/affective objectives; obtain multiple measures from multiple sources	Educational administrators, faculty
Accreditation/Certification Model	Faculty, administrators	Review content and procedures of instruction	Processes	Periodic points in time determined by accrediting groups	Discuss program, self-report, make professional judgments	Educational administrators; faculty accrediting groups
Stake's Countenance Model Client-centered evaluation	External evaluator	Report the ways different people see the program	Inputs, operations, outputs	Before, during after (immediately and later)	Describe what is intended in light of what is observed to have occurred, discover what audience wants to gather opinions	Public, content experts; faculty/clinical professional groups, students, etc.

Stufflebeam's CIIP Model Decision-oriented evaluation	External evaluator	Facilitate rational and continuing decision making	Inputs, operations, outputs, context	Before, during, after	Collect information needed by decision makers to assess the worth of the program	Administrators
Taba's Experimental-research evaluation	Researcher	Study cause and effect relationships to explain what works	Inputs, outputs	Before and after	Specify hypothesis and test utilizing experimental research design approach	Theorists, researchers
Scriven's Goal-Free Evaluation Consumer-oriented evaluation	External evaluator	Determine actual effects of a program, judge its merits	Inputs, outputs	Before and after	Gather data based on actual effects of program and assess impact of these effects on educational needs without knowing what goals had been specified	Administrators, faculty/clinicians

evaluating nursing programs, none are sufficient for accomplishing this task. All but one approach, that of the Accreditation/Certification Model, place responsibility for the evaluation with the external evaluator. The purposes for evaluating vary in each case but, with the exception of two (Scriven and Stufflebeam), do not explicitly identify decision making as a specific purpose that is reflected in the methods employed by the model. Only Stufflebeam focuses the evaluation on all program components and the context in which they occur. Regarding when to evaluate, only Tyler and Stake explicitly recognize the need to evaluate before, during, and immediately after the program, and later. Evaluation methods vary across models, with most favoring one approach over others that are available. None explicitly provide for balance in the types of methods, and only Tyler advocates the utilization of multiple methods within the context of the evaluation. Major audiences, for the most part, are limited in scope with the exception of Stake, who is very broad in his definition of audience.

In the absence of an approach for evaluating nursing programs that provides for the conditions specified earlier as necessary because of the nature of nursing and its settings, Waltz (Staropoli & Waltz, 1978; Waltz & Bond, 1982) developed an eclectic approach that incorporates the strengths of extant models. This approach also attempts to minimize limitations and expand thinking to include additional components and concerns with relevance to nursing education and service. During the decade following its development, the approach has been employed successfully by a variety of nursing programs in education and practice settings and has been refined on the basis of use. The components of Waltz's approach are discussed in the next section as they relate to evaluating programs in nursing education and service.

WALTZ APPROACH TO EVALUATING NURSING PROGRAMS

In this perspective, a *program* is defined as any ongoing activity that is designed to produce specified changes in the behavior of the individuals who are exposed to it (Astin & Panos, 1971). A program is an open system consisting of inputs, processes, and outcomes. *Inputs* into the program are affected by program processes and outcomes result. *Inputs* refer to:

1. The talents, skills, aspirations, and other potentials that the participants bring with them to the program.

2. Characteristics of participants' cultures, families, employing agencies, and nursing specialties.

3. Money, time, ideas, and resources available.

Processes include:

1. Program procedures and techniques; program content and substance; and styles of those who administer and implement the program, planned interventions, and strategies.

2. Environmental experiences, community and societal attitudes, and other psychological contexts in which the program is implemented.

Outcomes are:

1. Results as they relate to the attainment of goals and objectives.

2. Results as they relate to specific information needs of decisionmakers inside and outside the program.

The environment in which the program is planned, delivered, and evaluated is seen as salient in its own right, and how it affects and is affected by the program inputs, processes, and outcomes.

Evaluation is defined as a decision-making process that leads to suggestions for action to maintain and/or improve programs and participants' effectiveness and efficiency. For an evaluation to be considered successful, decisions must occur on the basis of the results, and, for this reason, decision making is considered during each step of the evaluation process. In this view, evaluation is distinguished from research per se. *Research* is conceived as a process of making decisions concerning statistical hypotheses and inductive inferences concerning the probable truth or falsity of a research hypothesis. Research results are generally not tailored specifically to the needs of decisionmakers, and, in most cases, the results of research are not immediately useful nor are they used in making decisions. Thus, the audience for research results is generally broad, including many who will not use the results. Research provides one paradigm for conducting a comprehensive evaluation of a nursing program, but, as noted earlier, this approach presents difficulty when used alone, if responsiveness is sought in the evaluation.

Similarly, measurement is not the same as evaluation. *Measurement* is a process of assigning numbers to objects to represent the kind and/or amount of a specific characteristic possessed by the object. It involves the regular and periodic collection of data upon which to base decisions and is a vital component of both evaluation and research; it constitutes the HOW of evaluation. In this approach to evaluation, many different measurement paradigms and methods are seen as appropriate depending upon the specific evaluation questions to be addressed.

The terms *decisionmakers* and *audience* are used interchangeably. The audience for evaluation consists of those individuals who will make decisions on the basis of evaluation results. Thus, audiences must be specified clearly during the planning stages of the evaluation, and then activities must be undertaken throughout with an eye to the information needs of the audiences, that is, taking into consideration the type of information upon which they will be willing to make decisions. In evaluating any given nursing program, there are a number of audiences both inside and outside the organization that must be taken into account. Potential *audiences* usually include individuals and groups who:

1. Plan or develop the program, including present and past planners, administrators, faculty and/or nursing staff.
2. Participate in the program, i.e., anyone who is directly involved in the implementation of the program in whole or in part such as faculty, students, and graduates in educational settings, and nurses and patients in practice settings.
3. Consume the products or services of the program. In educational settings, this would include, for example, employers of graduates, patients for whom students provide care; in the practice setting, examples include patients and their families.

In both settings, members of the profession and society at large, external funding sources, accrediting/certifying bodies, members of specific target groups, or communities would also be potential audiences for evaluation results. A particular audience may not be an audience for all activities conducted within the evaluation, however.

All nursing programs are viewed as having cognitive, affective, and performance components that must be considered in planning the evaluation. *Cognition* refers to subjects' theory and knowledge in regard to program content. *Affect* refers to subjects' attitudes, motives, and values. Affect is operationally defined as subjects' disposition to respond in a consistent manner to a certain category of stimuli (Campbell, 1963). *Performance* refers to subjects' psychomotor or behavioral skills that directly affect their nursing practice. *Confidence*, which is an affective component of particular interest in nursing, is viewed as specifically concerned with subjects' stimulation and self-assurance to take decisive action to implement their knowledge and/or to perform in a practice situation. A basic assumption is that while one may have sufficient knowledge, value the performance, and have the skill necessary to perform, nevertheless, one may or may not perform as a function of one's confidence, which should be considered as a focus for the evaluation.

Other aspects deserving consideration in planning for the evaluation include what Waltz refers to as supplemental activities and significant experiences as they relate to the conduct of nursing programs. *Supplemental activities* are those designed usually upon completion of the program to correct deficits or reinforce weak areas in the knowledge, affect, or skills of those who participate in the program. Perhaps the best examples of supplemental activities are the internships and extended orientation programs established by many service agencies in the last decade in an attempt to correct deficits, reinforce weak areas, and/or fill gaps in graduates' ability to practice nursing. Waltz advocates that by focusing on supplemental activities within the context of nursing program evaluations, such remedial work may occur in a more timely, appropriate, and relevant manner with less cost and that the products of nursing education, in this case, will be more marketable upon completion of the program. *Significant experiences* refer to those events occurring in the interval months between program and evaluation that may enhance or hinder the performance of subjects on evaluative measures. For example, it is not uncommon for graduates of nursing education programs and/or participants in continuing education programs to complete the program and then indicate on evaluative measures that a certain knowledge or skill, in their view, will be of little use to them in the practice setting.

However, later in the practice setting these same graduates often find themselves in a position to use this information because of new policies, procedures, or programs that are undertaken. Thus, this significant experience affects their view of knowledge or skill. At the time of the next follow-up of graduates, it will be reflected in their responses. The use of computers is an area where this is often seen, that is, graduates express no use for this knowledge and skill upon completion of an undergraduate program, then subsequently find themselves in a position where their employment setting converts to a data-based patient management system. If such supplemental activities and significant events are not taken into account in evaluating nursing programs, changes in programs could be made on the basis of evaluative data that might be premature and/or invalid, and the resulting changes ultimately might reduce the effectiveness of the program and/or increase its cost.

Table 2 summarizes the components of the Waltz approach to the

Table 2
The Waltz Approach to the Evaluation
of Programs in Nursing

WHO: *Internal evaluators, administrators, faculty,* and/or *nursing staff* as they implement evaluative responsibilities and functions inherent in their job descriptions.

WHY: *Make decisions re program and participant effectiveness* on an ongoing basis
   a) *Assess* extent to which *program and participant goals* and *objectives* are met
   b) *Answer questions of concern* to respective *audiences* (i.e., decisionmakers internal and external to the program)

WHAT: *Program goals and objectives, program inputs, processes, outcomes, environment participant cognition, affect, performance, audience questions*

WHEN: *Before, during, after* (immediately and later)

HOW: *Explicate cognitive, affective and psychomotor objectives* in behavioral terms; *identify questions of conern* to internal/external audiences; *employ unobtrusive multiple methods and sources* to obtain measures to assess objectives and obtain information useful to respective audiences in decision making; *provide balance* between objective-subjective measures; *utilize wide variety of study designs* ranging from purely descriptive to precise experimental including both qualitative and quantitative methods; *be cost efficient* by combining efforts and using what already exists whenever possible

   MAJOR AUDIENCE: *Planners, participants, consumers*

evaluation of programs in nursing. In terms of determining who is to be responsible for the evaluation, the approach recognizes the feasibility of using internal evaluators and for holding those within the organization accountable and responsible for the evaluation responsibilities that are part of their job descriptions. However, the importance of outside viewpoints are recognized, but their use is held to a minimum in order to contain the cost of evaluating. The primary purpose for evaluating is to make decisions regarding program and participant effectiveness and efficiency on an ongoing basis. Thus, decision making is paramount, and evaluation is both formative and summative in nature. The focus of the evaluation is upon the assessment of the quality of goals and objectives, as well as the extent to which they are met. Of equal importance is the focus on the need to answer questions of concern to various audiences. Concerted effort is made to elicit information regarding program strengths as well as weaknesses; to give equal attention during the planning stages to the importance and need for assessing inputs, processes and outcomes, their interrelationships with each other, and the environment in which they occur; and cognitive, affective, and performance components of the program.

Evaluation occurs before, during, immediately after the program, and later, using a variety of different methods and sources. Within the context of a given evaluation, there may be a variety of studies and evaluation activities occurring at the same and at different points in time conducted by individuals and groups, yet integrated by a Master Plan for Evaluation that is comprehensive in scope. This master plan is kept timely and relevant by an individual or group explicitly identified as being responsible for preserving the integrity of the Master Plan; coordinating the implementation of the evaluation activities contained therein; serving as a methodological resource to others involved in implementing specific activities; and managing the resources for evaluation with an eye to cost, quality, and methodological rigor. An attempt is made within the evaluation to use a variety of methods as appropriate, including, but not limited to, both qualitative and quantative methods, subjective and objective measures, and designs ranging from purely descriptive to experimental. Whenever possible, unobtrusive multiple methods and sources are used, and every attempt is made to use existing data sources in order to keep the expensive process of instrument development and testing at a minimum. Reliability and validity of instruments and other devices used within the context of the evaluation is a prime concern, given that results are to be used for decision making. Thus, only tools and measures demonstrating evidence for reliability and validity are employed. In addition, every effort is made to monitor and contain the cost for evaluating without sacrificing its comprehensiveness and the quality of the resulting decisions. Waltz and Bond (1985) contend that a comprehensive, yet cost-efficient, evaluation is more likely to result when the following occur:

1. A Master Plan for evaluation of the total program is developed on the basis of the information needs of the audience, and then specific evaluation efforts derive from this plan.

2. Evaluation is accomplished by holding individuals and groups accountable for evaluation responsibilities inherent in their jobs.

3. Dependence upon and the use of outside evaluators is minimized.

4. Evaluation efforts focus specifically upon the collection of information relevant to the needs of decisionmakers.

5. Evaluation focuses only on those behaviors critical to determining whether or not program goals and objectives were met.

6. Evaluators, whenever possible, employ instruments and other tools already in use for evaluation, and develop and test new tools only when essential.

7. The same tool or instrument is utilized to obtain similar information needed by several different audiences.

8. Tools and instruments employed for evaluation are specific, practical, reliable, and valid for the purposes intended.

9. A mechanism for directing information to the appropriate decisionmakers in a timely and relevant manner is established prior to the actual conduct of evaluation activities.

10. Priorities are established, shared with all involved, and then actually adhered to during the conduct of the evaluation.

11. Management techniques such as responsibility charting, Gantt charting, and engineering cost analysis are employed on an ongoing basis to maximize and monitor the efficiency of the evaluation process.

12. Provision is made for the ongoing evaluation of the evaluation, especially as it relates to the Master Plan.

In the final chapter, specific steps undertaken within the Waltz approach are discussed in detail. Specific strategies and techniques for implementing and managing the evaluation are also described.

SUMMARY

In this chapter, evaluation was defined as a decision-making process that leads to suggestions for action to maintain and/or improve effectiveness and efficiency of programs and participants. Purposes for evaluating nursing programs in education and service were explained. The principles that govern evaluation in nursing, which are the same as those that govern the evaluation of any programmatic endeavor, were presented. The unique and specific character of nursing and its settings, which must be taken into account when strategies and techniques for implementing these principles are designed and/or selected, were discussed. Of major concern was the selection of an approach to evaluating nursing programs. Models for evaluating programs that have served as prototypes for evaluation in a variety of settings and fields were presented. More specifically, the views addressed included: Tyler's Objective-Based Evaluation, Accreditation/Certification Evaluation, Stake's Client-Centered Evaluation, Stufflebeam's Decision-Oriented Evaluation, Taba's Experimental-Research Evaluation, and Scriven's Consumer-Oriented Evaluation. Also discussed was the Utilization-Focused Approach to Evaluation. However, while all prototypes contribute in some manner to the conditions necessary for conducting a comprehensive evaluation of nursing programs, none are complete or sufficient in this regard.

An eclectic approach to evaluating nursing programs developed by Waltz in an attempt to incorporate the strengths of existing models, minimize limitations, and expand thinking to include additional components and concerns with particular relevance to nursing was discussed. Attention was given to definition of terms, purposes for the evaluation, what the focus of the evaluation is, how the evaluation should proceed, when evaluation should occur, and major audiences. Specific considerations that increase the likelihood that an evaluation will be comprehensive but cost-efficient were elaborated.

REFERENCES

Alkin, M. C. (1969). Evaluation theory development. *Evaluation Comment, 2,* 2–7.

Ashburn, A. G. (1972). Directing education research training toward needs of large school districts. Texas A & M University, Texas (mimeo).

Astin, A., & Panos, R. J. (1971). The evaluation of educational programs. In R. L. Thorndike (Ed.), *Educational measurement,* 2nd ed. Washington, DC: American Council on Education.

Bloom, B. S., Englehart, M. D., Furst, E. J., Hill, W. H., & Krathwohl, D. R. (1956). *Taxonomy of educational objectives: Handbook I: Cognitive domain.* New York: David McKay.

Campbell, D. T. (1963). Social attitudes and other acquired behavioral dispositions. In S. Koch (Ed.), *Psychology: A study of a science, Vol. 6.* New York: McGraw Hill.

Campbell, D. T., & Stanley, J. C. (1963). Experimental and quasi-experimental designs for research on teaching. In N. L. Gage (Ed.), *Handbook of research on training.* Chicago: Rand McNally.

Cronbach, L. J., & Snow, R. E. (1969). *Individual differences in learning ability as a function of instructional variables.* Stanford, CA: Stanford University Press.

Cronbach, L. L., Ambron, S. R., Dornbusch, S. M., Hess, R. D., Hornik, R. C., Phillips, D. C., Walker, D. F., & Weiner, S. S. (1980). *Toward reform of program evaluation.* San Francisco: Jossey-Bass.

Floden, R. E. (1983). Flexner, accreditation and evaluation. In R. F. Madaus, M. Scrivner, & L. Stufflebeam (Eds.), *Evaluation models: View points on educational and human services evaluation* (pp. 261–278). Boston: Klumer-Nijhoff Publishing.

Glass, G. V. (1969). *Design of evaluation studies*. Paper presented at the Council for Exceptional Children Special Conference on Early Childhood Education, New Orleans.

Glass, G. V., & Maguire, T. O. (1968). *Analysis of time-series quasi-experiments* (U.S. Office of Education Report No. 6-8329). Boulder, CO: Laboratory of Educational Research, University of Colorado.

Green, L. W., & Lewis, F. M. (1986). *Measurement and evaluation in health education and health promotion*. Palo Alto, CA: Mayfield Publishing Co.

Guba, E. G. (1978). Toward a methodology of naturalistic inquiry in educational evaluation. *CSE Monograph Series in Evaluation*. Los Angeles, CA: Center for the Study of Evaluation.

Guba, E. G. (1976) *Alternative perspectives on educational evaluation*. Keynote speech at the annual meeting of the Evaluation Network, St. Louis, Missouri.

Hammond, R. L. (1972). Evaluation at the local level. Tuscon, Arizionia: EPIC Evaluation Center (mimeo).

House, E. R. (1980). *Evaluating with validity*. Beverly Hills: Sage.

Lindquist, E. F. (1953). *Design and analysis of experiments in psychology and education*. Boston: Houghton-Mifflin.

Madaus, G. F., Scriven, M. & Stufflebeam, D. L. (Eds.). (1983). *Evaluation models: View points on educational and human services evaluation*. Boston: Klumer-Nijhoff Publishing.

McDonald, B. (1975). Evaluation and the control of education. In D. Towney (Ed.), *Evaluation: The state of the art*. London: Schools Council.

Merriman, H. O. (1968). Evaluation of planned educational change at the local education agency level. Ohio: Ohio State University Evaluation Center (mimeo).

Metfessel, N. S., & Michael, W. B. (1967). A paradigm involving multiple criterion measures for the evaluation of the effectiveness of school programs. *Educational and Psychological Measurement, 27* (931–943).

Ott, J. M. (1967). A decision process and classification system for use in planning educational change. Ohio: Ohio State University Evaluation Center (mimeo).

Patton, M. Q. (1980). *Qualitative evaluation methods*. Beverly Hills: Sage.

Phi Delta Kappa Commission on Evaluation. (1971). *Educational evaluation and decision making*. Itasca, IL: Peacock Publishers.

Popham, W. W. (1975). *Educational evaluation*. Englewood Cliffs, NJ: Prentice-Hall, Inc., pp. 22–23.

Popham, W. J. (1969). Objectives and instruction. In R. Stake (Ed.). *Instructional objectives AERA Monograph Series on Curriculum Evaluation 3*. Chicago: Rand McNally.

Provus, M. N. (1971). *Discrepancy evaluation*. Berkeley: McCutcheon.

Reinhard, D. L. (1972). *Methodology development for input evaluations using advocate and design teams*. Unpublished doctoral dissertation, Ohio State University.

Rippey, R. M. (Ed.). (1973). *Studies in transactional evaluation.* Berkeley: Mc-Cutcheon.

Rutman, L. (1980). *Planning useful evaluations, evaluability assessment.* Beverly Hills: Sage.

Saylor, G., & Alexander, W. M. (1974). *Planning curriculum for schools.* New York: Holt, Rinehart and Winston, p. 8.

Scriven, M. (1983). Evaluation ideologies. In *Evaluation models* (pp. 229–260).

Scriven, M. (1974). Evaluation perspectives and procedures. In W. J. Popham (Ed.), *Evaluation in education—current applications.* Berkeley: McCutcheon.

Scriven, M. (1972). Prose and cons about goal-free evaluation. *Evaluation Comment, 3,* 1–7.

Scriven, M. (1967). The methodology of evaluation. In R. W. Tyler, R. M. Gagne, & M. Scriven (Eds.), *Perspectives of Curriculum Evaluation.* Chicago: Rand McNally. Reprinted in *Curriculum and evaluation,* A. A. Bellack & H. W. Kliebard (Eds.). Berkeley: McCutcheon, 1977, p. 645.

Stake, R. E. (1983). Program evaluation, particularly responsive evaluation. In G. F. Madaus, M. Scriven, & D. L. Stufflebeam (Eds.), *Evaluation models: View points on educational and human services evaluation* (pp. 287–310). Boston: Klumer-Nijhoff Publications.

Stake, R. E. (1976). *Evaluating educational programmes: The need and the response.* Paris: The Organization for Economic Cooperation and Development, pp. 20–28.

Stake, R. E. (1967). The countenance of educational evaluation. *Teachers College Record, 68,* 523–540.

Standards for Evaluation of Educational Programs, Projects and Materials. (1981). Developed by the Joint Committee on Standards for Educational Evaluation. New York: McGraw-Hill.

Staropoli, C., & Waltz, C. (1978). *Developing and evaluating educational programs for health care providers.* Philadelphia: F. A. Davis, Co.

Stufflebeam, D. L. (1969). Evaluation as enlightenment for decision making. In W. H. Beatty (Ed.), *Improving educational assessment and an inventory of measures of affective behavior.* Washington, D.C.: Association for Supervision and Curriculum Development, National Educational Association.

Stufflebeam, D. L. (1967, June). The use of and abuse of evaluation in title III. *Theory Into Practice, 6,* 125–133.

Stufflebeam, D. L. (1966, June). A depth study of the evaluation requirement. *Theory Into Practice, 5,* 121–134.

Stufflebeam, D. L. (1983). The CIPP Model for program evaluation. In G. F. Madaus, M. Scriven, & D. L. Stufflebeam (Eds.), *Evaluation models: View points on educational and human services evaluation* (pp. 117–141). Boston: Klumer-Nijhoff Publishers.

Stufflebeam, D. L., & Madaus, G. F. (1983). The standards for evaluation of educational programs, projects and materials: A description and summary. In G. F. Madaus, M. Scriven, & D. L. Stufflebeam (Eds.), *Evaluation models: View points on educational and human services evaluation* (pp. 395–404). Boston: Klumer-Nijhoff Publishing.

Stufflebeam, D. L., & Webster, W. J. (1983). An analysis of alternative approaches to evaluation. In G. F. Madaus, M. Scriven, & D. L. Stufflebeam (Eds.), *Evaluation models: View points on educational and human services evaluation* (pp. 117–141). Boston: Klumer-Nijhoff Publishers.

Suchman, E. A. (1967). *Evaluative research.* New York: Russell Sage Foundation.

Taba, H. (1966). *Teaching strategies and cognitive functioning in elementary school children.* Cooperative Research Project No. 2404; San Francisco State College, San Francisco.

Taba, H. (1962). *Curriculum development: Theory and practice.* New York: Harcourt, Brace and World.

Taylor, J. P. (1974). An administrators' perspective of evaluation. Michigan: Western Michigan University (occasional paper #2).

Tyler, R. W. (1949). *Basic principles of curriculum and instruction.* Chicago: The University of Chicago Press.

Tyler, R. W. (1942). General statement on evaluation. *Journal of educational research.*

Walker, J. (1974). *Influence of alternative, structural, organizational, and managerial options on the role of evaluation.* Paper presented at the Annual Meeting of the American Educational Research Association, Chicago.

Waltz, C., & Bond, S. (Eds.). (1982). *University of Maryland, School of Nursing Evaluation Packet.* Baltimore: University of Maryland.

Waltz, C., & Bond, S. (1985). How can an evaluation be comprehensive and yet cost efficient. *Journal of Nursing Education, 6*(24), 258–261.

Webster, W. J. (1975). *The organization and functions of research and evaluation in large urban school districts.* Paper presented at the Annual Meeting of the American Education Research Association, Washington, D.C.

Werner, W. (1978). Evaluation: sense-making of school programs, In T. Aoki (Ed.) *Curriculum evaluation in a new key* (p. 8). Vancouver: Center for the Study of Curriculum and Instruction.

Wiley, D. E., & Bock, R. D. (1967, Winter). Quasi-experimentation in educational settings: comment. *The School Review,* 353–366.

Worthen, B. R., & Sanders, J. R. (Eds.). (1973). *Educational evaluation: Theory and practice.* Worthington, OH: Charles A. Jones.

6

Evaluating the Program

Carolyn Feher Waltz

This chapter discusses specific steps undertaken within the Waltz approach, and strategies and techniques for implementing and managing the evaluation. As noted in the preceding chapter, a master plan for evaluation of the total program is developed on the basis of the information needs of the audiences, and then specific evaluation efforts derive from this plan. The implementation of the Master Plan is directed by an internal evaluator(s), who is responsible for maintaining the basic integrity of the plan, ensuring quality of action, coordinating participant efforts, and monitoring costs. The specific evaluation efforts deriving from the Master Plan are accomplished by those individuals and groups within the organization who are responsible for a particular activity. The primary purpose of evaluation is to provide necessary information to the appropriate decisionmakers in a timely and relevant manner. Therefore, management techniques such as responsibility charting, Gantt charting, and engineering cost analysis are employed on an ongoing basis by the evaluator(s) to maximize and monitor the efficiency of the evaluation process.

The specific steps undertaken in developing the Master Plan include:

1. Determining who will be ultimately responsible and accountable for the evaluation, who will be involved, in what manner, and to what extent.
2. Explicating why the evaluation is being conducted:

   a. stating the rationale for the evaluation.

   b. listing the purposes to be served by the evaluation.

3. Identifying the audiences for the evaluation and preparing a comprehensive list.

4. Determining what is to be evaluated:

   a. describing the program regarding inputs, processes, outcomes, and the environment.

   b. determining the focus for the evaluation.

      1. listing goals and objectives.

      2. explicating specific questions of concern to the audiences.

5. Determining how judgments will be made on the basis of evaluation findings:

   a. determining criterion standards for objectives.

   b. establishing and describing in written form a mechanism or procedure for making decisions on the basis of evaluation results.

6. Determining the activities that will be undertaken within the context of the evaluation:

   a. constructing a variable matrix that addresses evaluation questions, potential sources for answering each question, potential methods for measuring each question, and potential audiences for the result.

   b. summarizing and categorizing evaluation questions that have a common focus into sets of evaluation activities.

   c. determining evaluation activities that are being implemented, those under development, those conducted in the past, and those that need to be developed and implemented.

   d. determining who will be accountable and responsible for each evaluation activity.

   e. setting priorities in light of available resources.

   f. determining the cost to implement evaluation activities.

   g. determining when each evaluation activity will occur.

7. Establishing a system of reporting and record-keeping to ensure ready availability of evaluation results for decision making.

8. Establishing a mechanism whereby decisions made on the basis of results will be recorded and evaluated.

9. Establishing a mechanism whereby the evaluation effort and the Master Plan will be monitored and evaluated.

WHO WILL BE RESPONSIBLE FOR THE EVALUATION?

The Internal Evaluator

The individual(s) responsible and accountable for conducting the evaluation should be explicitly identified early. In a determination of who will be responsible for the evaluation, it is necessary first to appoint an evaluator(s) who will be ultimately responsible and accountable for directing the development and implementation of the Master Plan. Second, others who will be involved should be identified and the extent of their involvement considered. Third, it is important to identify and provide a mechanism for ongoing involvement of respresentatives of the audiences for the evaluation results.

Experience in evaluating a variety of nursing programs in varied settings suggests that an internal evaluator(s) can make continuous contributions to the development and maintenance of excellence in nursing programs. The evaluator can act as facilitator, researcher, mentor, linker, resource person, and change agent. Although there is concern that the evaluator's closeness to the program might interfere with objectiveness and create bias in evaluation, objectivity can be facilitated through the evaluative role and position within the organization. Utilization of an internal evaluator(s) has positive benefits that far outweigh any liabilities.

Establishing and Maintaining the Role

There has been much controversy about the usefulness of internal evaluators who are employed by the organization that is to be evaluated. A frequent criticism results from the ever-present potential for conflict of interest for the internal evaluator, since there is likely to be confusion about to whom ethical obligation is owed—to the organization paying for the evaluator's services or to the public to whom the organization provides services. It is clear that evaluations affect people in many ways and that evaluators are often at the mercy of political forces. Because of the political sensitivity of evaluation, Scriven (1975) proposed that it is important to confirm the evaluator's independence from what is being evaluated. When evaluators are employed by the organizations that are the object of their evaluations, it is often equally difficult to establish and maintain their independence as to control for possible bias.

In Waltz's view, program evaluation is conceived as an ongoing process integral with the operation of the nursing program. The Master Plan for Evaluation is a guide to the evaluation of all program aspects, addressing evaluative concerns of the respective audiences. The evaluators, who are internal to the organization, are responsible for ensuring that the plan is implemented, and the essence of the evaluation is determined on the basis of audience needs. Unlike other models, it is not determined by the evaluator, which reduces the influence of the evaluator in determining what will or will not be evaluated. Furthermore, the evaluators should not have operational responsibilities within the program that is being evaluated, but rather they should be directly accountable and responsible only to the program head (i.e., dean or director of nursing services). Also, they should be positioned in a separate unit that has been established solely for evaluation. In order for internal evaluators to operate effectively, proper organizational supports must be available. In this respect, the organization must perceive the internal evaluator's role as integral, and personnel and finances must be committed to the effort.

Nursing settings have several attributes that make them more amenable to internal than to external evaluators. First, there is a need for ongoing evaluative information. Administrators, faculty, and practitioners need this information on a regular basis if programs are to be delivered in the most effective manner; data regarding program inputs, processes, outcomes, facilities and resources, participants, and consumers all aid in decision making. In addition, monitoring changes in evaluative information is a monumental endeavor, but it is important. With external evaluators who move in and out of the system, continuity is not possible.

Second, evaluation is an expectation in all nursing settings. Nursing programs are required to maintain records about their programs, both in the immediate setting, and in the community and profession at large. Because evaluation is an integral part of nursing programs, it is an activity that is expected to occur on a routine basis as part of the job responsibilities of administrators, faculty, practitioners, and others. When such responsibilities are handed over to external evaluators, nurses are abdicating a vital part of their role. When internal evaluators are present, responsibilities and functions of administrators, faculty, practitioners, and others are facilitated by having someone continuously available to work with them in carrying out this aspect of their role.

Finally, administrators, faculty, practitioners, and others are faced with decision-making responsibilities in regard to policy making. Evaluation data should be readily available to aid in making decisions about almost all aspects of nursing programs. In the case of external evaluators, evaluation methods and the data they produce are not likely to be relevant immediately for the decisions required, especially in those instances in which evaluators complete their tasks and leave the setting prior to decision making. Information is needed that will guide decision making related to matters such as recruitment, retention, manpower needs, budgeting, needed program modifications, and, in some instances, justifying whether or not the program should continue. The lack of evaluation data can greatly thwart decision making in these areas and, most important, make the difference between proactive and reactive responses to the rapidly changing nursing and health care scene. Evaluation data should provide information to guide planned change as policy decisions are made. Internal evaluators are more likely to be sensitive to such changes and to collect evaluation data that will directly respond to these needs than are external evaluators.

Administrators at all levels of the organization should be convinced of the efficacy of internal evaluators and their contributions. They can help faculty, practitioners, and others in the organization understand the value of internal evaluators. The internal evaluator's role, when it is successfully implemented, should not remove others from responsibility for evaluation, but, rather, it should effectively facilitate their activities through systematic and planned data gathering and evaluation efforts. Administrators, faculty, practitioners, and others should be kept informed of and accountable for involvement in planned evaluation activities. Once appointed, the evaluators must include administrators and others in the process. With this continued interaction, all those involved stay attuned to the nature and scope of the evaluation that must be conducted.

Organization insiders need to be convinced that the evaluators' activities will be cost-effective financially and in utilization of personnel time. According to Waltz, evaluation efforts should be methodologically sound, but as cost-effective as possible. Care is taken to use established data sources, identify duplicative evaluation efforts, and plan strategies to reduce duplication. For example, in many settings grant-seekers collect the same type of information from the same individuals at different times, they are not aware that the data have been collected before. An internal evaluator aware of this could readily develop a plan in which the necessary data are obtained only once, then shared with those who need it. Similarly, in many educational settings, course evaluation data is collected by individual faculty with the cost in time and money required far greater than when a more coordinated and generalized approach is used. In one setting with which the author is familiar, the cost in faculty hours, secretarial time, materials, and computer time for 160 faculty to provide course evaluations by 1,000 students was five times greater than when a coordinated, schoolwide course evaluation was implemented. Since the use of an internal evaluator requires the commitment of financial resources, the organization must understand the potential contributions an internal evaluator can make. It must also be convinced that the establishment of the role is not only beneficial but cost-effective as well (Strickland & Waltz, 1981).

Operationalizing the Role

When the internal evaluator is part of the ongoing organizational structure, there are certain advantages for the operationalization of the role. Strickland and Waltz (1981) indicate that it affords the internal evaluator the opportunity to do the following:

1. Establish relationships with program personnel that exist over an extended period of time. An evaluator is more likely to be successful when there is rapport with important users (Alkin, 1980). When established relationships exist, there is potential for the evaluator to foster additional support from those within the organization in the implementation of evaluation activities. Another advantage stems from the fact that the evaluator can be called upon readily to facilitate related evaluation efforts that are within the domain of faculty or practitioners' responsibilities. However, a note of caution is necessary. There may be a tendency for administrators, faculty, or practitioners to "dump" unwanted tasks, for which they are responsible, onto the evaluator. Thus, it is essential that all be clear about situations when the limit of the role is to provide consultation and assistance rather than taking on a task that is more appropriately placed elsewhere in the organization.

2. Better understand the inner workings of the organization. As part of the organization, the internal evaluator is privileged to a more realistic and meaningful understanding of the day-to-day operations of the organization. This insight provides a better awareness of the resources, unique roles, idiosyncracies, and contributions of the pool of administrators, faculty, practitioners, and others. Such knowledge can enable the evaluator to plan more acceptable and appropriate strategies for implementing evaluation efforts. In addition, an understanding of the inner workings of the organization can facilitate more realistic interpretations of data and aid in formulating more practical recommendations when evaluation reports are provided. By being part of the organization, the in-

ternal evaluator can reiterate more readily important findings and encourage decisions to be made and implemented by the appropriate audiences.

Because of the ongoing nature of the internal evaluator's position and its special advantages, several functions have been found by Strickland and Waltz (1981) to be appropriate within the nursing setting, including: facilitator, linker, mentor, researcher, auditor, monitor, resource, and change agent.

Facilitator is a primary role, as the evaluator helps to frame evaluation questions based on audience input, then presents information that will aid in decision making. The evaluator also assumes responsibility for the development/implementation of selected program evaluation activities and works closely with program administrators, faculty, practitioners, and others to ensure that these activities reflect priorities and needs, including those of external audiences such as accrediting or certifying groups, legislators, and trustees. A major aspect of facilitation is dissemination and discussion of findings with appropriate audiences, both internally and externally, who have to make decisions about the program. Recommendations are formulated, and practical alternatives for action are drawn from the data that provide a basis for decision making. Decisionmakers are encouraged to use evaluation data as a basis for action.

The roles of mentor and researcher are taken on by the evaluator to aid individuals within the organization as well as committees and task groups. The evaluator designs procedures, collates information, and explains statistics and data to others during the evaluation. Much of the baseline information necessary for committees and task groups is provided by the evaluator so the groups may utilize more effectively the limited time they have to give to evaluation and decision making. The evaluator guides and works with others in accomplishing their tasks and provides leadership in many areas, particularly evaluation design and analysis. A major function of the evaluator is to teach others "how to" while working with them to develop more skills in evaluation and statistics. This activity also helps others to develop professionally and to conduct more competently their own research and evaluation activities.

As a monitor or auditor, the evaluator stays abreast of audience needs and assures that evaluation concerns are adequately addressed. The evaluator has responsibility for reviewing questions related to the program and modifying the Master Plan for Evaluation, since evaluation concerns change over time because of many factors inside and outside the organization. In addition, there is a need to monitor the results of program revisions made on the basis of evaluation findings. Most important, the evaluator monitors the cost and quality of the activities with an eye to the use of sound methods and practices.

A linker is "an individual who acts as a liaison between two or more subsystems in a communication system" (Guttentag, 1977, p. 332). As a linker, the evaluator helps to connect people within the program by communicating results between groups. The evaluator also serves as a link to the external world by identifying needs and priorities and ensuring that findings of evaluations are communicated to external groups. He or she communicates relevant evaluation findings from subsystems rapidly, in a manner that encourages greater use of results.

The evaluator serves as a resource to individuals and groups within the program as well as to the larger professional community. By actively consulting, publishing, providing continuing education, and being involved in other scholarly endeavors, the evaluator maintains credibility and objectivity and helps to reduce bias at the local level by providing a broader perspective.

Finally, the evaluator provides impetus for change in the organization. It is the responsibility of the evaluator to study the "efficacy of programs in accomplishing their appropriate goals" (Salasin, 1980, p. 6). The evaluator should use the program goals and audience needs as the major indicators to guide the direction of evaluation efforts. Major questions to be addressed include: (1) How well does this evaluation meet its stated objectives, especially as they relate to utilization of findings in decision making? (2) What factors, issues, and concerns inhibit the optimal accomplishment of these objectives? The reporting of data must be communicated often and on a regular basis to internal and external decisionmakers, and the evaluation plan must include strategies to ensure that these questions will be considered adequately. The evaluators serve as change agents by ensuring that the proper audiences receive the results of the evaluation efforts along with the evaluators' recommendations.

The evaluator should serve as a "judge" only in regard to methodology. That is, the evaluator must resist the tendency to become involved in decision making and instead remain in the role of provider of information to those who should make decisions; otherwise, the evaluator's objectivity and credibility may come into question. Appropriate judgments on the part of the evaluator relate to the selection, development, and employment of methodologically sound evaluation, measurement principles, and practices within the context of the evaluation.

Ethical and Political Aspects of the Role

Internal evaluators often face role conflicts that force the consideration of ethical and political aspects of their position. Evaluators employed on an ongoing basis in organizations are expected to conduct research facilitating operation of the program being evaluated. A potential political pitfall may occur if the evaluator is pressured to present findings and recommendations not supported by the data (Sieber, 1980) by those who seek to justify the program and its impact. The evaluator position can be a very powerful one, which is subject to abuse if the person filling the role is not ethical. This point is particularly relevant in the case of internal evaluators, who are likely to know more about the inner workings of the organization than others. Therefore, care must be taken by evaluators not to harm or "do disservice to their clients and to society through the improper and self-serving practice of their profession" (Stufflebeam, 1979, p. 5).

The role of the evaluator can potentially overlap with that of administrators, faculty, practitioners, or others. When an overlap does occur, its extent depends on the manner in which the evaluator chooses to exercise the role and the expectations of the organization. When extensive overlapping occurs, it can lead to conflict of interest and obligation that can result in harmful side effects for evaluation (Sieber, 1980). To avoid such dilemmas, it is important that participants be clear about the scope and limitations of their obligations to the program. It is the responsibility of the evaluator to remind others of these boundaries and to avoid exploitation of the position. He or she should know who is responsible inside the program for specific activities related to evaluation. Responsibility charting (Sloan, 1978), accomplished through negotiation, is a useful technique for communicating to others (a) who has veto power in regard to an evaluation activity; (b) who is ultimately responsible for its implementation; (c) who is expected to support the activity with manpower, materials, and money; and (d) who is to be informed of evaluation procedures and results. This management strategy is discussed and illustrated later in this chapter.

The politics that can surround the designing of evaluation activities, collection of data, and the interpretation and reporting of results can be sensitive. Results of evaluation efforts can have tremendous negative and positive affects on the program and its administrators and/or personnel. Possible consequences of a proposed mode of evaluation should be weighed carefully prior to implementation.

Internal evaluators have the advantage of being more likely to have a better awareness than external evaluators of the political forces operating within the program. This perspective is valuable because internal evaluators can be more knowledgeable about the organization's receptivity to specific evaluation strategies. Since program evaluation affects decision making and improvements within programs, the internal evaluators should devise approaches (e.g., co-aptation) that take the political forces within the organization into account but, at the same time, are credible and scientifically sound.

Confidentiality is also a sensitive concern. In some instances, lack of privacy, in the way that data is reported, can be harmful and jeopardize those involved in evaluation. Although it is not necessary to keep most program evaluation data confidential, care should be taken not to identify participants, particularly when this could be damaging. Participants' confidentiality must not be breached so that their input will be truthful.

A potential political disadvantage for internal evaluators is the danger of becoming scapegoats or for others to be made into scapegoats. If evaluators become too entwined in program operation and decision making, blame can be shifted more readily toward the evaluators when things go wrong or when conflict occurs. Care must be taken not to become part of known "political camps" within the organization, and evaluators must not be perceived as furthering professional goals through misuse of the position. Evaluation should be effected in such a manner that it serves the needs of the program and its participants in an unbiased manner.

The best approach to handling political concerns is to practice evaluation ethically, that is, when the evaluation plan is useful, valid, and efficient for the setting in which it is applied; when one communicates honestly with the audience for which data are gathered; and when results are reported in an appropriate, unbiased manner. Part of being ethical is to anticipate and circumvent conflicts of interest and to avoid unintended, harmful side effects of evaluation (Sieber, 1980).

Essential Characteristics of Internal Evaluators

While administrative support is a primary determinant of how successful internal evaluators may be in implementing their roles, the characteristics of those appointed to evaluator positions will also be important in determining the value of the roles. This author has found two attributes to be especially salient to the roles. First, evaluators must be skilled and knowledgeable. Competence in research design, statistics, measurement, and communication are necessary. As scientists, evaluators are expected to conduct valid research. This goal can only be accomplished when evaluators have good research background, education, and a broad repertoire of skills in using varied paradigms and evaluation methods. Within the nursing setting, the credibility of evaluation is influenced greatly by the evaluators' level of competence as perceived by the audience. It is also advantageous if the evaluators have expertise in the subject matter of the program under evaluation. Ability to communicate to audiences in unambiguous language at an understandable level is another important skill for evaluators.

Second, personal characteristics of the evaluators are important. Evaluators must be able to move about the organization freely and in a nonthreatening manner. They must possess personal integrity and, thereby, obtain the confidence of organization members. Not only must evaluators be politically astute, but they also must be willing to be flexible in order to involve people in evaluation activities. The ability to collaborate, and foster a positive attitude toward evaluation will complement evaluation efforts.

A word of caution is in order: Evaluation is, by nature, a threatening activity for most people, especially when it touches them personally. For this reason, it is not unusual for evaluators who have been perceived positively by organization members to suddenly be challenged when results begin to look less positive for the program or a particular individual or group. When this happens often, those who were most supportive of the evaluation effort become less so, and their discomfort manifests itself in challenges or criticisms of the evaluators or the evaluation methods employed. In such instances, it is important that the situation be looked at closely before support for evaluators or methods is withdrawn, or arbitrary, unwarranted changes in procedures are made. Internal evaluators, because of close association with the organization, are more vulnerable to this type of sociopolitical force, but it happens in the case of external evaluators as well.

Thus, the combination of administrative support, evaluators' knowledge, skills, and personal characteristics will determine their effectiveness.

Maintaining an Outsider Perspective in the Insider Role

It may become difficult for internal evaluators to maintain an objective stance over time when they are employed on a continuous basis by a program. For this reason, evaluators must question purposely and frequently whether involvement in the organization is biasing the evaluation. The evaluator should not become too involved in daily program operations or viewed as aligned with any organization, individual, or group. The evaluators must maintain some distance from the program that is the object of the evaluation. In this respect, they must not be accountable to the subjects of the evaluation. The key nursing administrator is the only person in the organization who should have approval or veto power for evaluation efforts, and it is to this individual the evaluators should be accountable. External evaluation consultants should be invited periodically to assist with the evaluation or to review certain aspects of the evaluation. This helps to bring an outside perspective to the effort.

When evaluation activities are designed, checks and balances should be built into the procedures to ensure that diversified viewpoints are taken into account. In this way, vested interests and biases can be cancelled out.

The step of determining who will be responsible for the evaluation effort is most important to its success. It is not sufficient simply to select someone in the organization to serve in this role because of availability, convenience, or interest, as is too often the case. Rather, great care should be taken to position evaluators effectively, with administrative support.

Determining Significant Others To Be Involved

Evaluation is most relevant when it involves people who will make decisions on the basis of results. Planners, participants, consumers, and the public, if they are potential audiences for the evaluation results, should have the opportunity to ask questions, and be involved in plan formulation, data gathering, outcome analysis, and conclusion decisions. If evaluation conductors and decisionmakers are kept separate, evaluation can become limited and irrelevant (Staropoli & Waltz, 1978).

Once the internal evaluators are appointed and administrative support is secured, attention turns to determining significant others to be involved, including: (1) those with evaluation responsibilities as part of their jobs, and (2) representatives of the audience. Program planners, participants, and the public are representatives of audiences most likely to make decisions using evaluation results. To secure the participation of these audiences, establish an evaluation committee or task force with representatives from each group. Such a committee should be viewed as a central coordinating body for evaluation activities but not as the group with the responsibility for conducting the evaluation. If evaluation efforts are to be comprehensive, they will require the involvement of many different individuals at varying levels of the organization, as well as those outside the organization. This cannot be accomplished by any one person or committee. In this respect, such a committee or task force may serve essentially three functions, including:

1. Bringing to attention efforts that are already in progress, so that they may become part of the overall evaluation.
2. Carrying communications regarding the progress of evaluation back to their respective groups.
3. Participating in the conduct of the evaluation by sharing ideas, needs, and resources.

These functions can be accomplished if the size of this group is kept small, and participation is based on interest and need for evaluation results. An advantage of the Waltz approach is its focus on the design of a Master Plan for Evaluation that incorporates varied evaluation efforts in such a manner that no one involved in the evaluation needs to be burdened with complete responsibility. Also, it is imperative that the tendency to include everyone at the early stage of the evaluation be halted or a precedent will be established for involving everyone at all stages of the evaluation. When this happens, not only does the evaluation process become unwieldy and costs escalate but interest and commitment of participants tend to wane. Only those individuals representing audiences who have specific information needs as a result of the evaluation should be members of the task force. In addition to the appointment of evaluators and a task force, it is necessary to identify responsible organization insiders.

It should be emphasized that there are as many vehicles for involving significant others in the evaluation as there are nursing settings. What has been suggested here, the committee or task force, is one such mechanism that often is used effectively in nursing. The important point is that in determining who is to be involved in the evaluation, provision must be made for the use of internal evaluators, involvement of respective audiences, and those inside the organization who have evaluation responsibilities as part of their job decriptions.

WHY CONDUCT THE EVALUATION?

Who Are the Potential Audiences?

Audience identification helps to clarify the reason for an evaluation. In Waltz's view, the primary purpose for evaluation is to make decisions regarding ongoing, program and participant effectiveness and efficiency. Specific purposes served by evaluation are listed in chapter 5.

In any evaluation, the purposes for evaluation are as varied as the individuals who are participating. For this reason, it is critical that time be given to answering the question, "Why has the decision been made ·to evaluate this program?" Is the evaluation occurring because accreditation is impending? Is evaluation occurring because people believe it is the thing to do? Are funding sources requiring it? Do those participating in the program seek directions for how to improve upon it? Is the concern with ascertaining whether or not the program subsequently effects changes in nursing practice? Is evaluation viewed as an objective means for resolving differences in opinions or professional debates?

The more comprehensive one can be during the planning stages, the more complete is the resulting Master Plan, and the higher the probability that it is relevant for the future. To determine priorities too soon may lead to a Master Plan that is too wide in scope, esoteric in view, and, ultimately, less useful for decision making. Thus, while not all purposes identified during the planning stages will be addressed when the plan is first implemented, it is important that one be as comprehensive as possible both in regard to the present and future.

Evaluation purpose will provide direction for methods designed at a later stage. For example, if a purpose is to obtain evidence upon which to base decisions regarding necessary program development and revisions, one may anticipate that evaluation methods will need to be both formative and summative, and that a more descriptive-type method (e.g., needs analysis) may be indicated.

As potential audiences become apparent, their needs and interests can be taken into account. In addition, it is possible that information deemed acceptable by one audience may not be satisfactory to another. For example, suppose a purpose for evaluation is to seek information regarding the efficiency of the program in terms of personnel time, and two audiences for results are program administrators and personnel. Staff members are interested in information regarding how their actual time involvement in the program compares with expected commitment, and its relation to their ability to carry out other aspects of their jobs. Although administrators are interested in this type of information, they also desire more specific data that allows them to establish justification for additional positions. What is acceptable data for personnel here is not adequate for the administrators' needs. However, the evaluation plan must provide for the collection of information that will satisfy the needs of both groups, in order to be successful. Often, this can be accomplished using one measurement method that elicits information needed—in this case, by both the administrators and personnel.

When a reasonably exhaustive list of purposes that reflect the views of planners, participants, consumers, and public is available, it should be reviewed to futher identify other purposes or potential audiences for evaluation results. The intent here is to identify additional purposes and audiences for the evaluation that may have been overlooked and to gain some indication of the relative importance of various purposes on the basis of size and importance of the audience.

Table 1 illustrates a list of potential audiences for results of evaluations of nursing programs in both educational and practice settings.

WHAT IS TO BE EVALUATED?

Evaluation focuses on assessing (1) the extent to which goals and objectives are met, and (2) answering questions of concern to respective audiences. It is useful to examine the program to ascertain what is known or unknown regarding inputs, processes, outcomes, environment, and their interrelationships.

The evaluation environment may affect the evaluation itself, as well as what is being evaluated. Generally, it is important to determine if the setting is stable and conducive to evaluation. Especially important to consider is if evaluation is likely to be sabotaged, or if it can be expected to function in a nonsupportive environment. Understanding and describing key elements in the setting promote a realistic evaluation effort and productive coexistence between evaluation and setting.

The setting also influences the object of the evaluation, and, for this reason, it is important to find out how elements in the setting, such as politics, economics, and social patterns, impact the program under evaluation. This is so that realistic interpretations of evaluation results can be made later. When the success or failure of a program or one or more of its respective components is reported, a piece of crucial infor-

Table 1
Potential Audiences for the Results of Nursing Program Evaluations

1. Program administrators (dean, director, vice president for nursing, associate and assistant deans)

2. Middle managers for the program (chairpersons, head nurses, nurse chairpersons, clinical coordinators)

3. Other administrators in the nursing setting who have programmatic responsibilities (directors of grants and funded projects, quality assurance coordinators)

4. Members of standing, ad hoc, and special committees

5. Past, present and potential faculty, clinicians, students, graduates and other staff

6. Professional associations and nursing organizations

7. Special interest groups (alumni associations, guidance counselors, recruiters, consumer awareness groups, other community special interest groups, political groups, news media, unions, etc.)

8. Accrediting, certifying, and licensing boards

9. Administrators and participants in other programs within the organization

10. Institutional administrators (president, chancellors, deans, chairs of other programs, etc.)

11. Federal, state, and local officials (governor, legislators, etc.)

12. Consumers and clients of the programs products (employers of graduates, competitive agencies; and institutions, patients, families, special target groups)

13. Collaborators (physicians, pharmacists, social workers, etc.)

14. Nursing programs in other educational and clinical settings

15. Funding sources (private donors, foundations, public sources, etc.)

16. Busybodies, friends, and enemies of the program or its participants

---

mation is the degree to which events in the setting were responsible. In a similar vein, should others wish to use the findings in another setting, they must determine the effect the setting had on overall results and judge its similarity to their own setting. In an evaluation that is ongoing and of large scope, it is essential that the setting be thoroughly investigated to decide whether the evaluation should be undertaken or, at a minimum, to prevent front-end problems in the design of the evaluation.

On the other hand, it is also important to determine how evaluation affects the setting. If the costs are too great, it is possible that the evaluation should be reconsidered, rescheduled, or relocated. If these are not options, then certainly the evaluation should be designed sensitively to respond to a hostile or unstable setting (Brinkerhoff, Brethower, Hluchyj, & Nowakowski, 1983). Environmental factors for consideration include organizational politics, program leadership, professional influences, history, organizational structure and climate,

Table 2
Questions of Concern in Regard to the Setting

Are there adequate resources available to support the program?
Are the necessary skilled personnel available and accessible?
Are the necessary facilities, time, and money available and accessible?
Is there access to the necessary support services and personnel?
Is there likely to be a change in resources that will affect the program or its evaluation?
How secure is the fiscal support system for the program and its evaluation?
Has a separate, adequate budget been allocated?
Will a written commitment of fiscal support be forthcoming?
Is the organizational climate supportive?
Is there political support for the program and its evaluation?
Are there opponents, proponents?
How secure is the program within the organization?
Who has formal and informal control over the program?
How do the program goals compare with goals of those within the organization who exercise control?
How supportive are professional groups of the program and its evaluation?
Are there special interest groups such as unions, and, if so, what is their agenda for the program and its evaluation?
How mature and stable is the program?
Has there been a history of self-appraisal and -evaluation?
Is the program stable enough to withstand evaluation?
What information regarding the program already exists?
How does the program fit within the larger organization?
What decisionmakers have potential to impact on the program?
What type of action or information by those with influence could jeopardize the program?
Is the program controversial in nature?
Are there legal restrictions that may impact on the program or its evaluation?
Are there professional organizational policies and procedures that may impact the program or its evaluation?
Is the program or its evaluation likely to be affected by any impending legislation?
What is the feasibility that an internal evaluator can function independently in the setting?
Is the setting conducive to evaluator/decisionmaker interaction?
Will it be likely that the evaluator will have access to the information necessary to answer key evaluation questions?
What kind of evidence is likely to make a difference in this setting?
Who will be influential in interpreting results?
Who is likely to influence the reporting of evaluation results, and what is the probable nature of that influence?
How much time is likely to be needed to manage the setting (e.g., is there political infighting, heavy administrative protocols)?
Will it be possible to bring in outside evaluators at critical points in time to lend credibility to the evaluation?
What characteristics must the evaluator possess to function most effectively in this setting?
(Staropoli & Waltz, 1978; Brinkerhoff et al., 1983)

economics, communication and social patterns, legal guidelines, and resources. Questions of concern in regard to setting are presented in Table 2. Methods of particular utility in investigating such questions include (1) conversations with key audiences, (2) conversations with specialists, (3) observations of the setting, (4) analysis of documents, and (5) interactions with existing groups. As a result of this examination, the following usually become apparent: (1) additional purposes to be served by the evaluation, (2) audiences that were overlooked in the foregoing step, and (3) what is unknown regarding program inputs, processes, outcomes, the environment, and their interrelationships, which should be addressed by the evaluation.

Next, goals and objectives should be scrutinized carefully. Program objectives establish criteria for evaluating the products or outcomes of the program, as well as its success. Thus, it is imperative that objectives be (1) realistic expectations for future behavior; (2) focused on changes in knowledge, attitudes, and performance that are to occur as a result of the program; (3) stated in clearly observable behavioral terms; and (4) stated so that crucial behaviors to be measured are evident and ranges of satisfactory/unsatisfactory performance in relation to these behaviors are apparent (Staropoli & Waltz, 1978, pp. 93–94). If it is evident that program objectives do not meet this criteria, they need to be refined before one proceeds further.

For those who require a review of how objectives may be stated so that they are readily measurable, Staropoli and Waltz (1978, pp. 152–155) and Waltz, Strickland, and Lenz (1984, pp. 165–167) may be helpful in this regard. In assessing objectives, it is also important to consider the link or lack thereof between objectives and expected outcomes, and between objectives and program processes. There should be a direct relationship between each objective, program processes designed to accomplish that objective, and expected outcomes. Too often, in the author's experience, program objectives have no counterpart in terms of program processes and, even more often, are not obviously related to expected program outcomes (Hart & Waltz, 1988). Each program objective should interface with institutional and organizational goals and have an explicitly stated counterpart among the goals and objectives for organizational subunits (e.g., departments, hospital nursing care units, courses, care plans, etc.). That is, program goals and objectives must be evident and directly related to their organizational counterparts.

In addition, it is helpful to consider audience goals and objectives by talking with representatives of each category (i.e., planners, participants, consumers, public). Consideration can be indirect as well, from written documents such as minutes of meetings and reports, published standards for nursing practice, grant proposals, newspapers, and institutional policies and procedures. At the same time, evaluation questions of concern to the respective audiences should be identified and recorded. It is useful, when one lists questions to be addressed by the evaluation, to categorize them according to focus, that is, questions that focus on inputs, processes, outcomes, participants, consumers, organizational structure, and environment. In this manner, it is possible to obtain some sense of balance or lack of it in the evaluations focus. For example, if the majority of questions focus on processes, and few on outcomes, given the importance of documenting that nursing makes a difference, one would probably seek additional outcome questions of concern to audiences and add them to the list. Also, by considering the size and importance of the audiences raising the same or similar questions, one is able at this stage to begin to prioritize questions that should be examined before others if resources are limited. Table 3 presents a lengthy list of questions that have been found to be of significance to audiences for the evaluation of nursing programs in a variety of settings over time.

HOW WILL JUDGMENTS BE MADE ON THE BASIS OF FINDINGS?

If evaluation is to be successful, then decisions must result from the findings in a timely and relevant manner. When possible, whatever process is employed for making decisions in the organization also should be employed for making decisions on the basis of evaluation data. Unfortunately, and too frequently, evaluations are undertaken with the assumption that the usual procedures for decision making will be employed and are known to all.

Typically, when findings are available, the discovery is made that, in fact, decision-making procedures are neither well defined nor well known. Precious time is lost in attempting to get data to the appropriate audiences while they are still timely and useful. The result, in most cases, is that by the time data are received by the appropriate audience, the decision has been made and the data are useful only in either validating or, in some instances, invalidating the decision that has already been made and implemented. For this reason, it is imperative that a procedure for decision making be clearly explicated during the development of the plan and shared with all concerned.

Two tasks are undertaken in planning for how judgments will be made on the basis of evaluation findings. First, it is necessary to deter-

Table 3
Questions of Significance to Audiences for the Evaluation of Nursing Programs

Are sufficient numbers of qualified applicants being recruited?	Is the program being selected by the most highly qualified of those accepted?	What do we know about participants' cognition in areas addressed by the program objectives prior to their involvement in the program?	What do we know about participants' skill in areas addressed by the program objectives prior to their involvement in the program?
What do we know re participants' attitudes in areas addressed by the program objectives?	What do we know of participants' general academic potential before involvement in the program?	Are requirements for program involvement realistic in terms of meeting the current needs of nurses in the state?	Are highly qualified faculty/clinicians attracted to the organization?
What is the responsibility of clinicians/faculty/administrators re the probationary period? (Who should determine needs, evaluate performances, make and implement the resulting decisions?)	Is the process by which participants are recruited reviewed? Is their involvement in the program effective and efficient?	Are support facilities and services adequate (e.g., office and work, laboratory and computing facilities, secretarial and clerical assistance)?	Is there adequate funding for the program?
Is there adequate funding for participants?	Is there adequate funding for faculty/staff development and research?	Are participants able to secure individual funding from external sources?	What are the educational experiences of participants in areas addressed by program objectives?
What are the educational experiences of participants in areas other than those directly related to program objectives?	What are the clinical experiences of participants?	What types of roles, if any, do participants assume in the profession of nursing?	Are participants doing research?
Are participants contributing to the evaluative efforts?	How and to what extent are participants involved in organizational activities (e.g., committee work)?	What is the level of job satisfaction (e.g., what blockages exist in the organization)?	What are the most important input factors in predicting success for participants?
What do we know of participants as they progress through the program?	What do we know of participants when they are involved in the program?	Are tools and other assessment of participants' performance reliable?	What participants are involved in the program?

Are participants' general academic potential before involvement related to the facility with which they implement the program?

What is the attrition rate?

What are the reasons for attrition?

What factors predict potential attrition?

What reasons do participants give for not continuing with the program?

How do participants judge the adequacy of the program?

Are participants satisfied with their program experiences?

Are participants satisfied with counseling and advisement?

Are participants satisfied with instruction available to them?

Are participants satisfied with consultation?

Do participants feel confident in incorporating program experiences into their ongoing practice during the program?

What contributions do participants make to the nursing and related literature?

Do participants provide leadership in formulating directions for health care locally, statewide, nationally?

Are areas of participant preparation, experience, and research expertise congruent with program objectives and responsibilities?

How effective are the participants in teaching others?

How effective are participants as clinicians?

How effective are participants as researchers?

How effective are participants as administrators?

How effective are participants as consultants?

Do participants use a diversity of activities in fulfilling their program responsibilities?

Are participants engaging in interdepartmental efforts?

What kind of service to underserved populations is provided by participants?

What is critical knowledge participants should learn in order to meet program goals?

Does the program provide the opportunity for participants to learn the expected skills and competencies?

Is the program adequate for meeting the needs of special populations (e.g., disadvantaged, elderly)?

Is implementation/involvement in the program smooth?

Are program activities sequenced appropriately?

Are specified prerequisites necessary and appropriate?

Is the program efficient in terms of resources, time, and cost?

Are the methodologies employed in the program appropriate for implementing the program?

Are the methodologies employed utilizing participant competencies to best advantage?

Are the methodologies employed facilitating job satisfaction?

Are the methodologies employed cost-efficient?

Does the program's approach to conceptualizing nursing facilitate high-quality nursing practice?

Does the program's approach to conceptualizing nursing facilitate the organization and delivery of nursing education?

Does the program's approach to conceptualizing nursing facilitate the conduct of nursing research?

Table 3 (continued)

Are objectives met through current clinical placement of participants?	Are objectives met through the current length of time of clinical experiences?	Are objectives met through sequencing of clinical experiences?	Do clinical facilities used for program implementation provide the clinical experience desirable for participants?
Are the needed clinical facilities available for participants?	Does the program articulate with the official position statements advanced by ANA, NLN, HEW, APHA, State Board of Nursing Examiners, Council of Graduate Schools, etc.?	How do the program components integrate into a total program beyond a series of activities the participant must successfully undertake?	Are program offerings comparable to those in similar institutions offering similar programs?
Does the program articulate with stated professional goals of participants?	Is the program responsive to the current and projected needs of society?	Does the program articulate with stated professional goals of participants?	How does workload relate to participant effectiveness?
How does workload relate to participant job satisfaction?	Does congruence exist among various participant expectations regarding collaboration in scholarly activity? What factors facilitate and limit such collaboration?	Does the program facilitate participant development?	Does the program facilitate the pursuance of advanced degrees of participation in postdoctoral learning activities by participants?
Is a high level of scholarly productivity maintained by participants?	Are there sufficient opportunities to allow stimulating, scholarly interaction among participants?	Does the administrative structure of the program facilitate effective and efficient operation?	Are collaborative relationships developed and maintained with other units of the organization and other individuals whose scholarly practice and/or research interests are supportive to nursing knowledge and practice?
Is there a reciprocal, enhancing, and developmental relationship between the organization and other agencies?	Have participants created an environment within the organization that allows participants to function?	Is duplication of efforts minimized across and within programs?	What is the formula whereby rewards are in direct relation to research, clinical, teaching, and service productivity and in which parity is assured across programs?
What type of organizational struc-	Is there an equitable exchange of	What are the most important	Is participants' general academic

ture is most effective for program goals and participants?

Do participants implement the program in the expected time?

Are participants satisfied with the consultations they received?

What kind of positions do participants take upon completion of the program?

What contributions do those who participated in the program make to the nursing and related literature?

What kind of service do underserved populations receive who participated in the program?

What do we know of participants' attitudes in areas addressed by program objectives after the program?

benefits between the organization and the individual?

How do participants judge the adequacy of the program after its completion?

Do participants feel confident in incorporating program activities into there ongoing practice after the program?

Are participants functioning in the roles for which they were prepared by the program?

Are subsequent employers satisfied with the level of competencies of those who participated in the program?

Are highly qualified participants retained?

Are those who participated in the program competent in carrying out program objectives as they provide ongoing nursing care?

through-put factors in producing success for participants?

Are participants satisfied with the counseling and advisement they received?

What supplemental or additional activities was it necessary for participants to seek after the program in order to reach their career goals?

What contributions to the nursing profession have come from participants?

Are consumers satisfied with the level of competency of participants?

What do we know of participants' cognition program objectives after the program?

Do we have evidence that those who participated in the program can and do collaborate in program planning and/or implementation with other health workers?

potential before involvement related to program completion?

Are participants satisfied with the instruction they received?

What significant activities do participants engage in after completing the program?

Do those who participated in the program provide leadership in formulating directions for health care locally, statewide, nationally?

Do employers need to provide additional experiences for those who participated in the program in order to facilitate their functioning?

What do we know of participants' skill in program objectives after the program?

What are the nursing practice characteristics of role models in clinical agencies employing participants?

Adapted from *University of Maryland School of Nursing Evaluation Packet*, C. Waltz and S. Bond (Eds.).

mine criterion standards for goals and objectives. Second, it is necessary to establish and describe in written form a mechanism or procedure for making decisions on the basis of evaluation results.

As noted in the preceding section, program goals and objectives must be stated in measurable terms, with criterion standards concisely included. The manner in which this may be accomplished is illustrated in Table 4, where selected goals and objectives operationalized during the strategic planning process at the University of Maryland School of Nursing are presented.

In identifying a procedure for decision making, one should keep in mind that in the Waltz approach, one method often is employed to obtain information needed by varied audiences and that not all of them will be audiences for all information generated by a particular evaluation method. This needs to be taken into account in whatever decision-making method is employed.

Decision-making rules are usually established in one of three ways: (1) by fiat, (2) by use of absolute standards, or (3) by group decision or consensus. Decisions made by fiat usually preclude successful decision making because they do not represent the views of all who are affected by them. When decisions are based on absolute standards, it must be possible to pinpoint crucial behaviors to be performed in relation to each objective, specify ranges of acceptable performance for each of these behaviors, and quantitatively measure the ability of individuals to meet the objective. Absolute criteria are the ultimate goal for any evaluation, since analysis of data in terms of absolute standards should automatically produce the decision. Unfortunately, absolute standards are difficult to establish for most of the objectives assessed by nursing program evaluations. A decision rule that may seem comprehensive when formulated in the abstract often fails in reality. The decisionmakers, when confronted with its implications, may be unwilling to accept the automatic decision. Thus, in the absence of norms or other rigid criteria, decisions are best determined on the basis of judgments made by committees or groups whose members represent the audiences for the result. As subsequent evaluation efforts are undertaken, and both content and methodology are refined, attention should be directed toward the identification of more precise, objective, and absolute standards, that is, the specification of what findings lead to what actions (Staropoli & Waltz, 1978, pp. 104–107).

Table 5 illustrates an example of a decision-making procedure employed by the University of Maryland School of Nursing that has proven its utility in other educational settings as well. The Delphi is an-

Table 4
Operationalizing Program Goals and Objectives—An Example

Goal	Operational Objective	Responsibility	Time Frame for Initiation
A climate and environment that facilitates and supports faculty research and scholarship activities	A. Acquire the services of a grant writer	Director, research center	January 1984
	B. Increase efforts to obtain peer review of scholarly work	Individual faculty	January 1984
	C. Increase research and reference books in health sciences library and research center reading room	Individual faculty, directors and chairs	January 1984
	D. Increase numbers of faculty involved in interdisciplinary seminars, conferences, and other activities that foster interdisciplinary research	Department chairs and faculty, assistant dean for continuing education	March 1984
	E. Provide workshops and consultations on publishing scholarly papers for faculty and students	Assistant dean for continuing education, director, research center, and individual departments	June 1984
	F. Appoint additional faculty to the research center	Dean	July 1984
	G. Provide private offices for all senior faculty	Dean	August 1984
	H. Establish policies regarding routing and approval mechanisms for research proposals/activities, reimbursement for research-related activities and related matters	Dean	September 1984
	I. Make computer facilities in the research center available for use and staff on an expanded basis	Assistant dean for academic services and director, research center	September 1984
	J. Increase submission of proposals for external funding	Faculty	Fall 1984

Adapted from "University of Maryland School of Nursing, Long Range Goals," Spring 1983. Working document.

Table 5
Decision-Making Procedure—An Example

The University of Maryland School of Nursing is a large, complex organization in which judgments are made according to a matrix model for decision making. To facilitate the efficiency with which the findings resulting from this evaluation are used to make decisions, it is necessary to adopt a procedure for making judgments that recognizes that different types of evaluative information may be useful to different individuals making decisions at different levels of the organization and that a given set of evaluation findings may be of concern to a number of different audiences. Therefore, it is recommended that the following procedure be employed for making judgments on the basis of the findings from this evaluation.

1) Prior to the development of a specific evaluation activity, the evaluator(s) will collaborate with the appropriate administrator(s) in order to identify all the potential audiences for the findings likely to result from the implementation of the activity.

   A. Activities that are implemented schoolwide require collaboration with the dean, the associate dean for undergraduate studies, the associate dean for graduate studies, the assistant dean of continuing education and faculty development, the assistant dean for academic services, and the director of the doctoral program.

   B. Activities that are specific to the undergraduate program require collaboration with the associate dean for undergraduate studies (or designee).

   C. Activities that are specific to the master's program require collaboration with the associate dean for graduate studies (or designee).

   D. Activities that are specific to the doctoral program require collaboration with the director of the doctoral program (or designee).

   E. Activities that are specific to the continuing education program require collaboration with the assistant dean of continuing education and faculty development (or designee).

2) The methodology for this evaluative activity then will be developed and implemented under the direction of the evaluator(s), taking into consideration the needs of each potential audience. In this manner, the probability is increased that the evaluation will provide the type of information upon which the respective audiences are willing to base decisions.

3) When the evaluation data are obtained, a report of the findings organized in terms of the evaluation questions will be compiled and considered by the evaluator(s). The evaluator(s) will make recommendations for action and will identify questions to be added and/or deleted during subsequent evaluative efforts.

4) The findings and recommendations will be forwarded to the appropriate administrator(s) (see no. 1), who will subsequently identify in collaboration with the evaluator(s) those individual(s) who will render decisions on the basis of the evaluation findings. The administrator(s) will also suggest additions and deletions in evaluation questions to be addressed by later evaluative efforts.

5) The report, including recommendations for action, then will be presented to the appropriate audience(s) by the evaluator(s).

6) Decisions will be made and implemented by the audience(s). Notification of actions taken on the basis of evaluative findings and suggestions for questions to be addressed by subsequent evaluative efforts will be forwarded to the evaluator(s) by the audience(s) rendering the decision.

Adapted from *University of Maryland School of Nursing Evaluation Packet*, C. Waltz and S. Bond (Eds.), University of Maryland, 1982.

other approach that may be useful in situations in which it is not possible to bring members together for meetings or when knowledge of others' views may confound group decisions, for example, in situations where power struggles may dominate group process and influence decision making. This indirect method allows participants to respond to the arguments of others without subjecting them to possible extraneous social pressures. When this approach is used, it is possible to determine the following: (1) some idea of the degree of consensus behind the overall group decision, (2) opinions and preferences of specific subgroups, and (3) revisions in opinions and stated reasons for why they occurred (Helmer, 1966; Staropoli & Waltz, 1978; Waltz, Strickland, & Lenz, 1984). The Delphi technique and modifications of it have been employed by institutions to establish program priorities and resource allocations (University of Maryland Strategic Plan, 1986), by those who establish policy (Moscovici, Armstrong, Shortell, & Bennett, 1978) and by those seeking to establish priorities for the nursing profession (Lindeman, 1975; Ventura & Walegora-Serafin, 1981).

In summary, whatever procedure or mechanism is selected for making decisions on the basis of evaluation findings, it should be described in written form during the planning process, before any data is collected, and it should be made known to all involved.

HOW WILL THE EVALUATION PROCEED?

Several tasks are involved in determining the activities that will be undertaken within the context of the evaluation. It is necessary to:

1. Construct a variable matrix that addresses questions, potential sources for answering each question, potential methods for measuring each question, and potential audiences for the result.
2. Summarize and categorize evaluation questions that have a common focus into sets of evaluation activities.
3. Determine which activities are already being implemented, under development, conducted in the past, and need to be developed and implemented.
4. Determine who will be accountable and responsible for each evaluation activity because of their job.
5. Set priorities for implementation in light of resources available.
6. Determine the cost of implementing evaluation activities.

Constructing the Variable Matrix

The variable matrix is a valuable mechanism for planning an evaluation that will be comprehensive in scope; balanced in focus; employ multiple, varied methods and sources; and provide specifically for the information needs of the audiences. It is also a very useful vehicle for communicating to others the nature and substance of what will occur within the context of the evaluation. A sample variable matrix appears in Table 6.

In construction of the matrix, it is first necessary to reorganize the evaluation questions to be answered. This is done to provide the information needed by audiences for decision making in categories reflecting whether they refer to program inputs, processes, or outcomes. For indexing purposes and to facilitate updating of the matrix, all input questions are designated by a 1 and then sequentially numbered, all process questions are designated by a 2 and then sequentially numbered, and all outcome questions are designated by a 3 and then sequentially numbered. In this manner, it is possible to tell at a glance whether a particular question refers to inputs, processes, or outcomes, as well as to add with ease new questions as they arise. Theoretically, it is possible to add numbers ad infinitum (although this would not be feasible for practical reasons), simply by adding 11, 22, or 33 and sequentially numbering as necessary. Because the evaluation should be tailored to decision making, there may well be instances in which it is no longer useful or necessary to seek answers to a given evaluation question, since the results are no longer of interest to the audience. In such cases, this indexing system allows one to retire a question without forfeiting its number or place in the matrix. At some future time, if it is necessary to reconsider the question, it can be retrieved with ease.

Next, for each evaluation question, it is necessary to identify all possible sources for obtaining answers to the question. Again, the intent here is to be as comprehensive and exhaustive as possible during the planning stages. Ultimately, when resources allow, multiple sources then may be employed in answering a given question, and responses may be compared for consistency or inconsistency. When consistency among several different sources exists, then evidence for validity of findings is strong. Inconsistencies often provide useful direction for areas requiring further study or for necessary improvements in the program.

Suggested methodologies for measurement are identified for each question. Again, with an eye to the use of multiple methods to answer

Table 6
A Sample Variable Matrix

Question Inputs	Potential Data Source	Suggested Methodologies	Potential Audiences
101. Are sufficient numbers of qualified applicants being recruited?	Students, faculty, administrators, written documents	Survey, interview, audit review of documents	Administrators, legislators, faculty, federal funding agencies, students-peer groups, graduates, clients, accrediting groups
102. Is the program being selected by the most highly qualified of those accepted?	Student, faculty, administrators, written documents	Survey, interview, audit review of documents	Administrators, faculty, legislators, students, graduates, clients, peers, accrediting groups, federal funding agencies
OPERATIONS			
201. What do we know of students' cognition as they progress through the program?	Students, faculty peers	Objective test, students perceptions, review of products, peer surveys, faculty surveys, grades, etc.	Faculty, administrators, students
202. What do we know of students' skills as they progress through the program?	Students, faculty consumers, written documents, peers	Performance simulation exercises, review of products and written materials, survey of consumers, patients, peer surveys, interviews, critical incident technique	Faculty, administrators, students
OUTPUTS			
301. Are students' general academic before admission related to program completion?	Students, written documents	Correlation of general academic potential variables, student characteristics with program	Administrators, faculty, students, graduates, accrediting groups
302. Do students finish in the expected time?	Students, written documents	Survey, time analysis, review documents	Administrators, faculty, students, graduates, accrediting groups

Adapted from *University of Maryland School of Nursing Evaluation Packet,* C. Waltz and S. Bond (Eds.), University of Maryland, 1982.

any given question, the intent is to be as comprehensive in scope as possible. Also, in identification of possible methods of measurement, attention should be given to the following: use of existing methods and secondary sources whenever possible, as opposed to undertaking tool development and testing, which is very costly; employment of unobtrusive methods; balance of the types of methods utilized, so that both subjective and objective measures are proposed; utilization of a wide variety of different types of methods in addition to the usual paper and pencil measures; and use of the appropriate type of measure for the type of data desired.

Measurement is the process of assigning numbers to objects to represent the kind and/or amount of an attribute possessed by them (Waltz et al., 1984). *Instrumentation* is the process of selecting or developing devices and methods appropriate for measuring the criteria established for making decisions in relation to an evaluation problem (Staropoli & Waltz, 1978, p. 111). Tools and other measuring devices can be classified by (1) what they seek to measure, (2) the manner in which they are constructed and interpreted, (3) the type of respondent performance they seek to measure, and (4) who constructs them. Table 7 summarizes each of these types of measures.

In evaluating nursing programs, three types of measurement devices are of particular interest: those that seek to measure cognition, affect, and performance. *Cognitive* instruments are used to assess accomplishment of objectives before and after the program or to assess participants' knowledge and understanding of the content addressed by the program as it is implemented. Indicators of status of change in cognitive behavior include:

1. Achievement tests (objective and essay) that measure the extent to which cognitive objectives are attained.
2. Self-evaluation measures designed to determine participants' perceptions of the extent to which cognitive objectives are attained.
3. Sentence completion exercises designed to categorize the types of responses and to enumerate their frequencies relative to specific criteria.
4. Rating scales and checklists for judging the qualities of products produced in conjunction with or as a result of the program.
5. Interviews to determine the frequencies and levels of satisfactory responses to formal and informal questions raised in a face-to-face setting.

Table 7
Types of Measures
Classification for Tools and Other Measuring Devices

Construction and Interpretation	What Is Measured	Types of Respondent Performance	Who Constructs Them
Norm-referenced—respondents' performance is evaluated relative to performance of others in some well-defined group; measure is designed to maximally discriminate among subjects possessing differing amounts of attributes measured	*Cognition*—seek to assess subjects' knowedge or achievement in a specific content	*Maximum performance*—interest is in assessing participants as they do their best (i.e., produce their highest quality work); usually are indices of cognitive behavior	*Standardized*—developed by specialists for wide use; content is set, directions for administration and scoring are prescribed; norms information concerning scores is generally available
Criterion-referenced—respondents' performance is evaluated relative to a set of well-defined criteria or target behaviors; measure is constructed to discriminate between subjects who have and have not acquired the target behaviors	*Affect*—seek to determine interests, values, and attitudes *Psychomotor skills*—seek to measure participants' ability to perform specific tasks, carry out specific procedures, techniques, etc. *Physical functioning*—seek to quantify the level of functioning of living beings	*Aptitude*—tests of specific measures of capacity for success and tend to focus on various general aspects of human ability *Achievement*—are more specific than aptitude and tend to measure particular skills and knowledge *Diagnostic*—focus on even more specific skills and often employ multiple measures of a particular skill; intent is to pinpoint weaknesses that might not be apparent otherwise	*Informal*—developed by the examiner for own use; content is not constrained, examiner is free to determine administration and scoring procedures; norms usually are not available
Objective—allow participants little if any latitude in constructing their response and prescribe scoring criteria *Subjective*—allow considerable latitude in responding; probability that different people score differently is greater		*Typical performance*—are measures of affective behavior and usually attempt to have respondents describe the way they typically perceive themselves or their behavior; usually ask forced choice responses, or criterion-keyed responses	

6. Peer utilization surveys to ascertain the frequency of selection or assignment to leadership or resource roles.

7. Questionnaires employed to determine the frequency of responses to items in an objective format or number of responses to categorized dimensions developed from the content analysis of responses to open-ended questions.

8. Anecdotal records and critical incidents to ascertain the frequency of behaviors judged to be highly desirable or undesirable.

9. Reviews of records, reports, and other written materials (e.g., articles, autobiographical data, awards, citations, honors) to determine the numbers and types of accomplishments of participants (Staropoli & Waltz, 1978, pp. 111–112).

Affective measures seek to determine interests, values, and attitudes. It is difficult to preserve the conceptual differences between interests, values, and attitudes when one is actually constructing measures of affect. Thus, in order to render them measurable, they are all subsumed under the rubric of acquired behavioral dispositions (Campbell, 1963) and are defined as tendencies to respond in a consistent manner to a certain category of stimuli. Indicators of status or change in affective behaviors include:

1. Self-report inventories designed to yield measures of adjustment, appreciation, attitudes, interests, temperament, etc., from which inferences can be made concerning the possession of psychological traits (e.g., defensiveness, anxiety, confidence).

2. Sentence completion exercises designed to obtain ratings of the psychological appropriateness of an individual's responses to specific criteria.

3. Interviews.

4. Questionnaires.

5. Semantic differential, Q sort, and other self-concept perception devices.

6. Physiological measures.

7. Projective techniques (e.g., role playing, picture interpretation).

8. Observational techniques and behavioral tests, including measures of congruence between what is reported and how an individual actually behaves in a specific situation.

9. Anecdotal records and critical incidents.

Performance instruments seek to measure respondents' ability to perform specific tasks, to carry out specific procedures, techniques, and so forth. Criteria for the behaviors to be assessed must be stated clearly. Task analysis procedures are often used for this purpose (Gagne, 1962). Direct and indirect observation methods are most viable to this type of measurement.

The two major frameworks for measurement are norm referenced and criterion referenced. *Norm-referenced* measures are employed when the intent is to evaluate a subject's performance relative to the performance of others in some well-defined comparison group. Criterion-referenced measures are used to compare a subject's performance with a well-defined set of criteria or behavioral tasks. Depending upon which of the two approaches are employed, the specific procedures for tool development and testing will vary.

Objective instruments contain items that allow respondents little, if any, latitude in responding and specify criteria for scoring so clearly that scores can be assigned by individuals who know little or nothing of the content. Multiple-choice tests are good examples of instruments with a high degree of objectivity. *Subjective* instruments allow the respondent considerable latitude in responding. The probability that different scorers may apply different criteria in scoring is greater here. Case studies are good examples of subjective measures.

An important consideration in regard to evaluation methods is that they demonstrate reliability and validity. *Reliability* refers to the consistency with which a tool assigns scores to a group of respondents. Factors affecting reliability are (1) the manner in which the instrument is scored, (2) the characteristics of the measure itself, (3) the physical and/or emotional state of respondents at measurement time, and (4) the properties of the situation in which the measure is administered (e.g., noise, lighting conditions). If an instrument does what it is intended to do, that is, if it is useful for the purposes intended, it is said to have *validity*. Both reliability and validity are matters of degree. Each time an instrument is used, its reliability and validity should be assessed to ensure that it is behaving as planned. Not only should instruments employed within the evaluation demonstrate these characteristics, but the whole process of measurement is more apt to be reliable and valid if multiple measures of the same element are employed. That is, more than one type of instrumentation is employed to answer any given evaluation question. Multiple-measures use increases the probability that the evaluation results will be more reliable, valid, and useful. Those readers desiring more information on measurement and or the various types of instrumentation available will find the works by Staropoli and Waltz (1978); Waltz and Bausell (1981); and Waltz, Strickland, and Lenz (1984) useful for this purpose.

Methods aimed at assessing monetary costs of programs should be given special attention in selecting and/or developing methods for addressing evaluation questions. Especially in periods of fiscal austerity, evaluations that fail to address costs do a disservice to decisionmakers. Thompson, Rothrock, Strain, and Palmer (1981) note that a program with substantial benefits in excess of risks may represent an unwise societal choice if costs are exorbitant; a program with relatively limited benefits may be a wise investment if net costs are negligible. Thus, cost data must be obtained within the evaluation and, ideally, should include consideration of overall costs and how they will vary with possible program modifications. While elaborate cost analyses may not be feasible, basic aggregate figures can still provide valuable guidance. Thompson et al. emphasize that no program or program component can be justified unless its benefits exceed its costs. This principle must be applied to cost analysis itself, that is, the method of cost analysis employed for program evaluation should not overshadow the likely benefits to decisionmakers. Thompson et al. also compare alternative approaches to cost analysis that may be useful for those planning to use such approaches within the context of the evaluation.

Finally, for each evaluation question, all potential audiences for results are identified.

Advantages of this Variable Matrix Approach to delineating the evaluation questions include:

1. Directing attention to the relationship between the evaluation questions and the program components (i.e., inputs, processes, outcomes), thus facilitating the identification of gaps in areas to be investigated by the evaluation.

2. Suggesting potential data sources and when data collection should occur, thus giving some indication of the relative demands to be placed on those who will participate.

3. Demonstrating the types of methods that may be used to render each question measurable, thus stimulating consideration of tools and methods that are currently available, those that need to be developed, and the extent of the work to be undertaken.

4. Stimulating thinking about the next step of the process and evaluation methodology, thus preserving the necessary relationship be-

tween determining what is to be measured and how it is to be rendered measurable.

5. Preserving the necessary relationship between activities undertaken within the context of the evaluation and audience information needs.

When the matrix has been constructed, it is wise to elicit input and reaction to its contents from organization insiders who are responsible for implementing evaluation activities, and from others in the audience.

Categorization of Evaluation Activities

Questions in the variable matrix that are similar in focus are categorized into sets of evaluation activities, as demonstrated in Table 8. In the table, each activity is named, and the index numbers of the questions in the variable matrix that comprise the activity are specified in parentheses in the second column. This step reduces the many evaluation questions to a more manageable amount for those who have to assume responsibility for further development and implementation. In addition, when others assume responsibility for a particular activity because it is part of their job descriptions, they are able to move directly from the Categorization of Activities to the Variable Matrix, where they are provided with specific questions to be addressed by the activ-

Table 8
Categorization of Evaluation Activities—An Example

Activity	Variable Matrix Evaluation Questions
1. Students evaluation of curricular components: a. Courses b. Clinical experiences c. Specific learning strategies and techniques d. Methods of evaluation of student performance	(203, 211, 212, 213, 214, 215, 222, 229, 230, 231, 232, 233, 234, 235, 236, 238, 239, 240, 241, 242, 243, 244, 245, 246, 250, 251, 252, 273)
2. Students appraisal of faculty performance	(212, 213, 214, 218, 220, 221, 222, 223, 224, 264, 265, 270)
3. Graduate evaluation of the curriculum as a whole	(303, 304, 305, 306, 307, 309, 310, 312, 313)
4. Graduate evaluation of curricular components	(303, 304, 305, 306, 307, 309, 310, 312, 313)

Adapted from *University of Maryland School of Nursing Evaluation Packet*, C. Waltz and S. Bond (Eds.), University of Maryland, 1982.

ity, potential sources, methods, and audiences for results. In this manner, they are able to fulfill their responsibilities without deviating from the Master Plan, but without having the burden of being intimately familiar with the whole plan.

Assigning Responsibility for Evaluation Activities

When completed, the evaluation activities listed in the Categorization of Evaluation Activities should be scrutinized to determine the following: (1) activities already being implemented in some manner; (2) activities under development; (3) activities conducted in the past; and (4) activities not under development, not in place at present, and that need to be developed and implemented. Identification of individuals and groups who are contributing (or have done so) is important. Usually, activities under development or in place can serve as prototypes for activities within the Master Plan. Typically, activities undertaken prior to the systematic program effort are more narrow in scope than those needed to meet the information needs of the audiences, but they can readily be expanded to provide needed additional information. Another rich source of methods is what is developed informally by others in the organization for their own needs or interests. These are often not widely known because they have been developed as working-type documents. When such methods are shared, they can help in meeting current evaluation needs.

Job descriptions of those in the organization, as well as descriptions of policies and procedures of task forces and committees, and minutes of important meetings (e.g., staff meetings), should be scrutinized to identify those organization insiders who have responsibility for evaluation activities in the Master Plan. When the evaluators have a good sense of who should be responsible for evaluation activities, they should then meet with administrators to discuss planned activities to facilitate additional identification of responsible parties.

Efficiency in an operation is defined as producing effectively with a minimum of waste, expense, or unnecessary effort. The extent to which this is achieved in the evaluation of nursing programs is largely a function of how four interrelated factors—accountability, relevance, timeliness, and communication—are managed. Cost in regard to accountability for the evaluation, that is, determining who is to be responsible and answerable for evaluation activities, is a major concern (Waltz & Bond, 1985, p. 258). If individuals and groups inside the organization are held accountable for evaluation responsibilities, not only can the cost for evaluation be reduced considerably, but evaluation also becomes an ongoing aspect of the day-to-day operation. The ultimate purpose for evaluation, decision making, is apt to occur more efficiently.

Accountability for evaluation activities occurs at all levels of the organization. Therefore, accountability must be formally assigned and communicated to all participants to prevent duplication of effort. This can be accomplished by employing a relatively simple management technique developed by Sloan (1978), referred to as *Responsibility Charting*. Table 9 illustrates such a responsibility chart. The process of responsibility charting involves identifying what is to be accomplished (in this case, evaluation activities from the Categorization of Activities) and listing them on the left of the chart vertically (row headings). Across the top of the chart (column headings) are listed those inside the organization who are involved in the evaluation. Sloan offers classifications or levels of commitment that are negotiated and placed in the appropriate cell of the chart. "A" signifies approval/veto, and the individual with the "A" has ultimate approval or rejection authority. As suggested earlier, in nursing settings where internal evaluators are employed, the "A" is usually granted only to the key administrator for the nursing program. "R" represents responsible; the individual with the "R" has responsibility for implementation of the designated activity. Responsibility cannot be shared, although activity may be delegated, and only one individual can have the "R" for an activity. In the case in which a task force or committee is actually responsible for an activity, the chairperson should be given the "R," to eliminate confusion. "S" signifies support; this individual must provide support and resources to the possessor of the "R" for the particular activity. These must be provided unless institutional resources are not sufficient to support the commitment, in which case a request must be made for additional commitment of these resources at a higher level of the organization. Finally, "I" signifies informed; it designates the individuals who are to be kept informed of what is happening in the evaluation effort. They can comment or attempt to persuade those who possess the "R" if they disagree with the activity, or if they feel changes are indicated in procedures but do not have veto or alteration power.

Responsibility charts are useful at all levels of the evaluation process. While the example is for a programmatic application, the charts are helpful in delegating steps in the procedures for implementing a particular activity (Table 10).

Responsibility charts are most effective when all involved are present

Table 9
Responsibility Charting—A Programmatic Application

Evaluation Activity	Dean (1)	Coordinator for Evaluation (2)	Evaluator BSN (3)	Evaluator MS (4)	Evaluator PhD (5)	Associate Dean-Undergrad. (6)	Associate Dean-Grad. (7)	Assistant Dean-CE (8)	Asst. Dean-Acad. Service (9)	Director Doctoral Program (10)	Director Research Center (11)	Dept. Chairpersons Undergrad. (12)	Dept. Chairpersons Grad. (13)	Evaluation Comm. Undergrad. / Evaluation Comm. Graduate (14)	Doctoral Program Comm. (15)	Director Media Center (16)	Asst. to Dean for Acad. Serv. (17)	Faculty BSN (18)	Faculty MS (19)	Faculty PhD (20)	Faculty CE (21)
1. Direct the implementation of the revised Master Plan	A	R	S	S	S	S	S	S	S	I	S	I	I	I	I	S	S	S	S	S	S
2. Communicate with significant others including chairpersons, departments, key committees (curriculum, doctoral program, continuing education) regarding the activities of the Office of Evaluation.																					
3. Obtain and file reports and other written documents that pertain to evaluation activities within the Master Plan.	A	R	S	S	S	S	S	S	S	S	S	S	S	I	I	S	S	S	S	S	S
4. Place responsibility for developing and implementing activities in the Master Plan where they belong by virtue of job/committee functions and responsibilities.																					
a. Continuing Education within program activities	A	R	S	S	S	S	S	S	S					I	I						I
b. BSN within program activities	A	R	S	S	S	S	S	S	S			I		I	I			I			
c. MS within program activities	A	R	S	S	S	S	S	S	S				I	I	I				I		
d. Doctoral within program activities	A	R	S	S	S	S	S	S	S				I	I	I					I	

Key: A, Approval/veto; R, responsible; S, support; I, informed.
Selected portion of the University of Maryland, School of Nursing Responsibility Chart for 1982-1983, Working Document, Office of Evaluation.

Table 10
Responsibility Chart For Implementation Of An Evaluation Activity (Sample): The Program Assessment Questionnaire (PAQ), (Steps 4 and 5)

Activity	Coordinator for Evaluation	Evaluator, BSN	Evaluator, MS	Evaluator, PhD	Evaluation Research Analyst	Evaluation Secretary	Doctoral Research Assistant
Steps							
4 (a) Analyze quantitative data	A	S	S	S	R	S	S
(b) Construct tables	A	S	S	S	R	S	S
(c) Interpret data	A	S	R	S	S		
5 (a) Prepare initial report in accordance with Master Plan	A	S	R	S	S	S	
(b) Type initial report	A		S			S	
(c) Proofread initial report	A		R			S	
(d) Distribute initial report to appropriate audiences	I	I	S	I	I	R	
(e) Present initial report to appropriate audiences	I	I	R	I	S	I	

Key: A, Approval/veto; R, responsible; S, support; I, informed.
Selected portion of the University of Maryland, School of Nursing Responsibility Chart for 1983-1984, Working Document, Office of Evaluation.

when responsibility delegation is determined. This is especially true within organizational units when participants work as a team to determine responsibility; job functions become more clearly defined, and the unit works cohesively.

Responsibility charts not only define accountability, but they also serve as communication tools for informing others about evaluation activities that are underway and for clarifying the roles of individuals involved in the activity both inside and outside the unit. Responsibility charting reduces interunit conflict as well as unit-organizational conflict, and it is useful in resolving debates. Their existence precludes the possibility of personnel denying responsibility for a task's completion. If responsibility charts are utilized as working documents, the result will be a savings in the total cost of the evaluation effort (Waltz & Bond, 1985, p. 259).

Determining the Cost of Evaluation Activities

The budget for evaluation is the plan for acquiring and using financial resources to conduct the evaluation. Knowing the anticipated and actual costs for the specific activities within the plan is a great help. Generally, the evaluation budget contains the following items:

1. Personnel (salaries and fringe benefits)
2. Consultants
3. Travel and per diem
4. Printing and postage
5. Conferences and meetings
6. Data processing
7. Supplies and materials
8. Overhead (space, utilities, telephone)
9. Equipment

Brinkerhoff et al. (1983) suggest as a rule of thumb, that an evaluation budget should be approximately 10 percent of the program or project budget when a one-shot evaluation will serve short-range and focused program needs only. As with all rules of thumb, they note that this is simply a starting point and that evaluation can also be budgeted at 15–25 percent when evaluation is ongoing. Brinkerhoff et al. also note the importance of accurately estimating costs associated with various evaluation tasks so that plans for needed resources can be made. Of particular concern in costing out evaluations are (1) the type of information collected; (2) the amount of information needed; (3) the location of information sources; (4) the timeline; and (5) the cost of personnel involved in collection, analysis, and reporting. Provisions made during the planning stages of the evaluation promote fiscal accountability in the evaluation as it is implemented and later evaluated. Brinkerhoff et al. suggest that this accountability is promoted when evaluation context provides for:

1. Maintenance of accurate financial records with public access.
2. Consideration of cost alternatives and comparison shopping or contract bidding for goods and services.
3. Documentation of changes in the design or environment that bring about budgetary adjustments.
4. Accounting for dollars spent on evaluation objectives and tasks.

5. Systematic review of the budget in light of evaluation progress.
6. Inclusion of fiscal information in interim and final reports for the public record (p. 190).

Because of the large number of individuals and groups who are ultimately involved in implementing activities contained in the Master Plan, mechanisms must be put in place to monitor the cost of each activity. A technique that has proven useful in this regard is *Engineering Cost Analysis.* The purpose of such an analysis is to break down costs to the smallest cost component. For example, when the cost of typing a form is being researched, this should be broken down into number of pages and cost per page. In addition, all costs associated with the activity should be included (i.e., costs for materials and manpower time). It is useful to include administrative, faculty, practitioner, secretary, data analyst, and research assistant time as appropriate in order to monitor how much total personnel time is necessary for completion of the activity. Table 11 presents a completed engineering cost analysis for an activity where items have been broken down into initial and continuing costs. This breakdown is particularly appropriate for this type of activity, since it is the first implementation of a planned, ongoing activity. Cost analysis highlights the cost of the initial expense of the activity as compared to the estimated costs of following implementations. Therefore, the cost/benefit of placing ongoing activities is apparent. This example also depicts the breakdown costs to the smallest-unit-cost component. For example, typing is broken down per page, and personnel time is broken down per hour.

In the subsequent cost analysis for the ongoing activity, it will be useful to build the learning curve effect into the costs. This effect is simply the improvement in productivity that results from experience. For example, the data analysis for this activity will be a less time-consuming task when it is implemented the second time, since the data analyst is now familiar with the procedure and computer program. Also, faculty time will be reduced in the analysis and reporting of data, since protocols will have been established.

Another example of engineering cost analysis is an approach used to examine alternatives. In Table 12, the following alternatives are presented: (1) administer both forms to all respondents, (2) administer one form to all respondents and the second form to 30 percent of the respondents, and (3) employ only one form for all respondents. The analysis assists in realizing the costs involved as the length of a form is increased. For example, in this case there is a $253.30 difference be-

Table 11
Engineering Cost Analysis for an Activity
with Initial and Continuing Costs—The Course Evaluation
Questionnaire (CEQ)

Initial costs[a]		
200 Faculty Guidelines (3 pages)		
Typing	$1.25/page	$3.75
Xerox	$0.045/copy/page	$27.00
2,000 Student directions (1 page)		
Typing	$1.25/page	$1.25
Xerox	$0.045/copy/page	$90.00
2,000 CEQ forms A,C		
Typing	$1.25/page	$2.50
Xerox	$0.045/copy/page	$90.00
2,000 No. 2 lead pencils $0.32/dozen		$53.33
Subtotal for initial costs		$267.83
Continuing costs		
2,810 Optical mark reader cards (based on Fall, 1981: 825 enrollment in MS and PhD courses and 1,985 enrollment in BSN courses)		
	$6.00/1,000	$16.86
COMPEVAL	$111/computer hr[b]	$50.00 (est)
SPSS Run Time	$111/computer hr	$10.00 (est)
Analysis and report of data—data analyst time		
20 hr	$7.10/hr	$112.00
Faculty Time—10 hr	$10.55/hr[c]	$105.50
Subtotal for continuing costs (est)		$294.36
Spring 1982 total costs (initial and continuing)		$562.19

[a]Faculty time in pilot study report preparation was not included to avoid duplication of costs.
[b]Computer time should not be confused with clock time.
[c]Based on an average graduate faculty member's salary.
Taken from Hutchins, E., Arnold, E., Cogliano, J., Parelhoff, S., and Wolfe, M., In C. Waltz and S. Bond (Eds)., *Course evaluation. University of Maryland School of Nursing Evaluation Packet.* University of Maryland, 1982.

tween using both forms and only using one form, while there is a $73.79 difference between using both forms and using both forms with 30 percent sampling for the second form. Naturally, prior to making a decision, other factors must be considered, such as response rates and benefit analysis, especially in regard to decision-making information provided when both forms, rather than one, are used.

This analysis also demonstrates that there are certain costs that do not increase as the quantity of respondents increase. All the starred items indicate that these costs are not inflationary as the size of the sample and the response rate increases. This is useful to know, as the

Table 12
Engineering Cost Analysis of Alternatives to Administering
the Alumni Survey

	Across and Within Forms to All Graduates ($)	Across Form to All and With 30% Sampling for Within Forms ($)	Across Forms Only to All Graduates ($)
Paper	10.00	8.00	6.00
Envelopes	5.00	5.00	5.00
Postage	40.00	40.00	40.00
Key punching	32.00 (2 hr @ .16/hr)	23.00 (1½ hr @ .16/hr)	16.00 (1 hr @ .16/hr)
Computer analysis of data	100.00	80.00	50.00
Preparation of questionnaire for mailing	73.95 (15 hr)	59.16 (12 hr)	49.30 (10 hr)
Typing and distribution of reports[a]	98.60 (20 hr)	98.60 (20 hr)	73.95 (15 hr)
Assistance with report writing by data analyst[a]	56.00 (10 hr)	56.00 (10 hr)	28.00 (5 hr)
Faculty time for report writing and directing tasks	200.00 (20 hr)	200.00 (20 hr)	200.00 (15 hr)
Estimated total	811.55	737.76	558.25

[a]Cost of these items would remain the same regardless of the number of alumni surveyed and should only be included for the first 100 graduates surveyed when costs are estimated.

Taken from Strickland, O., Fontaine, D., Booth, R., and Vore, A. In C. Waltz, and S. Bond (Eds.), *Alumni survey, University of Maryland School of Nursing Evaluation Packet*, University of Maryland, 1982.

size of the subject pool grows and questions about the expense of administering to all subjects arise. A word of caution is necessary: Engineering cost analysis is useful to the degree of accuracy of the estimation of costs. Costs estimated for the amount of time a task takes must be monitored; those involved must keep records of their actual time.

Engineering cost analysis is a tool for increasing the efficiency of the evaluation process, because efforts that are expensive relative to their benefits can be identified and remedied. It also serves as a communication tool, when necessary, to identify how the budget was allocated and/or to justify the budget for evaluation.

Establishing Priorities for Evaluation Activities

It has been emphasized throughout that comprehensiveness in planning is essential so that the resulting Master Plan will well serve the program for many years. When the evaluation plan is implemented, however, it is critical that priorities are established for the varied activities in the plan. It is neither feasible nor possible to implement all activities in the plan at any given point in time. Real-world constraints, as well as audience needs, require that certain activities be ongoing, that others be implemented only once, and still others at periodic points in time. An important consideration, once the evaluation activities have been identified, is the determination of priorities.

As noted earlier, priorities should be established on the basis of several considerations:

1. The size and importance of the audience in need of information generated by a particular evaluation activity.
2. The availability and/or willingness of individuals to take on the investigation of a particular activity.
3. The strengths and weaknesses of the individuals who take on evaluation activities in the areas of research, evaluation, measurement, and the content addressed by the activity.
4. The amount of time available to the individual or group designated as responsible for a particular activity.
5. The availability of others to help with the activity.
6. The support services available to the individual responsible for the activity (e.g., research assistance, consultants).
7. The money available for evaluation (i.e., cost of an activity, in light of total budget, for evaluation).
8. The cost to respondents to serve as sources of data for an activity, and the effort/cost required to obtain the data needed to conduct a particular activity.
9. The availability of computers, computerized literature searches, etc.

10. The availability of instruments and/or secondary data sources in regard to the activity.

11. When the information elicited by the activity is needed by the decisionmakers.

12. The extent to which the activity contributes balance to the evaluation (i.e., objectivity/subjectivity needed, a varied paradigm).

WHEN WILL THE EVALUATION OCCUR?

In evaluating nursing programs, usually, both summative and formative evaluation activities are involved. Formative approaches are used in those instances in which information is collected to provide immediate feedback to improve the program and/or participants' effectiveness. When formative evaluation is undertaken, certain considerations need to be made in determining when activities will be implemented during the conduct of the program. For example, it is necessary to consider the following: when, during the program, participants will benefit most from an assessment of program strengths and weaknesses and from a profile of progress in meeting objectives; when will audiences be ready to accept findings from the program evaluation activities that are different from what they would like to see; and when will audiences be willing to make the necessary changes in the program before it is completed. One must also look at whether evaluation should occur as part of the ongoing program activities or at specific points that are separate from regular operations. It is generally less costly to evaluate in conjunction with regular program operations, but when this approach is used, data may be subject to social influences that affect the validity of the decisions made, for example, participants may be threatened that unfavorable responses will affect their ongoing relationship with those responsible for the program.

On the other hand, evaluation that is separate from program operations may produce more valid decisions, but there is a danger that it will not continue to be viewed as vital to the ongoing program. The decision on when to evaluate should be made only after consideration is given to all possible effects of the evaluation, positive and negative, in terms of what is currently occurring in the program. Times selected to evaluate should be least disruptive to the ongoing program.

Summative evaluation occurs upon completion of the program. Here the concern is in terms of when after the program it is most advantageous to collect information. It is necessary to take into account intervals of time between evaluations that allow for identification of supplemental activities and significant experiences; how much time must lapse before information is available to answer the evaluation questions of concern (e.g., how long does it take for program learnings to be incorporated into practice?); and the length of time audiences are able to wait for evaluation results to be obtained.

Relevancy refers to the degree to which the evaluation is related to the matter at hand; an evaluation that is not relevant cannot be cost-efficient. When dates for the completion of various evaluation activities are defined, effectively communicated, and adhered to, availability of data for decision making is apt to be more timely. If utility of evaluation findings is to be enhanced and cooperation and support are to be elicited, it is a must that the effective exchange of evaluation information occur and that evaluation timetables and procedures be communicated and understood at all organization levels (Waltz & Bond, 1985, p. 260).

Gantt Charting, exemplified in Table 13 and developed by Henry J. Gantt, can be especially useful in this regard. It is a management technique designed to show planned progress for a number of activities displayed against a horizontal time scale. The chart is useful in depicting schedules and capacities of faculties, personnel, and resources. The activities to be accomplished and the individual responsible are listed vertically on the chart, with the applicable time period appearing across the top of the page. As with responsibility charts, Gantt Charts can be used programmatically, as in the example, and they are also useful within the context of specific activities. Utilizing the Gantt Chart, the administrator can visualize how the different activities relate to each other in terms of time, cost, and resource allocations.

Gantt Charts can be used to map out the steps of a particular evaluation activity, the sequencing of the steps, and the resource and time requirements for each step. As a control tool, the planned Gantt Chart, compared to what actually occurs, will provide red flags as to where breakdowns and/or bottlenecks occur in regard to a particular activity. Gantt Charts, as responsibility charts, are best used when all those involved are present when the chart is developed. Those who actually perform the activities are best qualified to estimate the time each activity requires. It should also be noted that Gantt Charts should be revised, as experience dictates that an activity actually takes less or more time than currently indicated on the charts.

The most important function of the Gantt Chart is its ability to keep the evaluation effort timely. But the charts can also serve as tools for

Table 13

Gantt Charting: A Programmatic Example for Accomplishment of Across Program Activities (2-month interval),[a] January/February

Activity	Month											
	January	February	March	April	May	June	July	August	September	October	November	December
1) Analyze fall CEQ forms	R											
2) Administer minimester CEQ forms to students	C											
3) Report 9-month fall alumni survey to executive committee	X											
4) Analyze data fall PAQ-S		R										
5) Report PAQ-F to executive committee		O										
6) Report of fall CEQ forms to individual faculty		C										
7) Analyze minimester individual CEQ		R										

Personnel Responsible for Activity: C, coordinator for evaluation; X, evaluator PhD; O, evaluator MS; R, evaluation research analyst.

[a] Selected portion of the University of Maryland School of Nursing Gantt Chart for 1982–1983, Working Document, Office of Evaluation.

prioritizing both evaluation activities and the steps within a given activity. Having a visual document of scheduling and resource requirements of an activity utilized in combination with the known benefits of the activity, it is possible for one to identify those activities that indicate the lowest cost with the most benefit to the evaluation effort. By utilizing Gantt Charts, responsibility charts, and engineering cost analysis in combination, it is possible to keep the links of the evaluation effort in unison when, as in most evaluation operations, there is a physical separation of personnel and resources.

REPORTING AND RECORDING

When evaluation involves many different individuals inside and outside the organization, as it does in this approach to evaluation, it is imperative that (1) a system of reporting and recording be established to ensure ready availability of evaluation results for decision making, and (2) a mechanism be established whereby decisions made on the basis of results are recorded. Most important, the Master Plan for Evaluation should be available in written form and easily accessible by those involved in the effort. The components of the plan should include:

1. A statement of who is responsible for the evaluation, others involved, and the nature and extent of their involvement.

2. A list of purposes to be served by the evaluation.

3. A comprehensive list of potential audiences.

4. A list of goals and objectives stated in measurable terms.

5. A procedure for how decisions will be made on the basis of evaluation findings.

6. A variable matrix containing evaluation questions, potential sources for answering each question, potential methods for measuring each question, and potential audiences for the results of each question.

7. A list of evaluation activities to be undertaken with the questions to be addressed by each activity indexed by number to the variable matrix.

8. A responsibility chart identifying who is accountable and responsible for all activities on the list of activities.

9. A programmatic timetable identifying when each activity on the list of activities is to occur.

10. Guidelines for preparing evaluation reports and for recording evaluation decisions.

11. Procedures for evaluating the evaluation and a timetable for when they are to be implemented.

12. Sample forms to be used in the conduct of evaluation activities by individuals and groups by virtue of their jobs, as follows:

    a. protocol guidelines

    b. responsibility chart

    c. engineering cost analysis form

    d. Gantt Chart

In addition, for each activity undertaken within the context of the evaluation, there should exist a manual that includes items a–d above. If the evaluation is to be long-lasting, it is imperative that procedures be recorded so that those new to the organization can be readily oriented to the effort and that the responsibilities of those who leave the organization can be readily assumed by their replacements.

Since many different audiences will need information contained in evaluation reports in whole or in part, it is necessary to develop a standard approach to the preparation of reports. This will allow easy access to those portions of reports required by different audiences. It is important that the name of the activity, as listed in the categorization of activities, and the variable matrix index numbers for the question addressed always be included on the title page of the report. The report contents should be organized around the evaluation questions, and results should be presented as responses to the questions. Since most information requests from audiences are in the form of questions, when this format is used it is relatively simple to extract the appropriate questions and their responses from the report in order to meet the request quickly. Each time a report is prepared, attention should be given also to the procedures used to obtain the information, to the reliability and validity of the tool used for this, to information generated by the tool that may no longer be relevant, and to information needed that is not generated by the tool, but requires addition of questions to the tool and/or the Master Plan.

In the section of the report immediately following the presentation of findings, options for action emanating from the data should be listed. Evaluation reports should be as concise as possible. For parsimony, procedures for obtaining the data should be described in full in the first report for a specific activity, and in subsequent reports only deviations from protocol (and their justification) should be reported.

Reports should be available in a central place, usually the evaluation unit, and they should be filed by activity and questions addressed, for easy access. Whenever possible, a computerized system of indexing and/or reporting should be used. Experience has demonstrated that it is costly and inefficient to provide copies of reports to others within the organization for information only; instead, full reports are best supplied only to those audiences who will need the findings for decision making. Availability of reports in a central, easily accessed place is generally sufficient for interested non-decisionmakers. It should be noted that, in some instances, reports may contain confidential and/or sensitive information that may be shared only on a need-to-know basis. For this reason, it is usually best to note on the title page of the report whether the report contents are open to anyone or, if not, to list those who may access. In extremely confidential cases, it is best to require a view request from the individual or group responsible for the activity.

Brinkerhoff et al. (1983) suggest that a report plan be devised describing how information will be shared with key members of the audience. They note that a good reporting plan can contribute greatly to the value of the evaluation by assuring that audience members are provided the opportunity to tell those who conduct the evaluation whether or not the information is timely, understandable, believable, and useful. Table 14 presents an example of a report plan using the format suggested by them.

Finally, it is necessary to establish a mechanism whereby the actions taken on the basis of the results are recorded. There are many different ways to accomplish this readily. In some cases, a standard form is employed, to be completed by the appropriate audiences, then placed in the central file. In other instances, copies of written documents; (e.g., minutes, where the decisions are recorded) are forwarded by the audience for inclusion in the central file. The most important consideration in selecting the means to accomplish this is that the method be palatable and easy for audiences to use. Since decision making is the expected outcome of successful evaluation, one cannot assess whether or not the evaluation is effective if the outcomes of the evaluation process are not known.

EVALUATING THE EVALUATION

Meta-evaluation, evaluation of the evaluation, involves assessing evaluation efficiency and effectiveness in the three following areas: (1) the Master Plan, (2) the implementation of the evaluation plan as a whole

Table 14
Sample Report Plan

Activity	Audience	Content	Format	Frequency
Course evaluation questionnaire	Faculty	Summary statistics for their own student responses to the questionnaire, means and variances for all courses and for courses similar to their own, reliability statistics	Printout from SPSS program runs	One month after completion of courses each semester via interdepartmental mail
Program assessment questionnaire	Faculty, administrators, students	Summary statistics for present administration, graphs to compare findings across previous two years, changes noted in both positive and negative direction	One page written summary, overhead transparencies, oral presentation at faculty meeting attended by above audience representatives	Yearly during December faculty assembly

Adopted from a format suggested by Brinkerhoff et al., 1983.

as well as each of the specific activities within the plan, and (3) strategies and techniques for managing the evaluation. It should be evident from the preceding discussion that provision is made during the planning and implementation stages of the evaluation for those involved, as well as for audiences, to evaluate the evaluation on an ongoing basis.

1. During the planning stages, opportunities for reaction and input are provided to those involved, as well as to the audiences.
2. The process of plan development is such that it is imperative at each step.
3. Strategies and techniques, such as the variable matrix, are designed to allow the results of assessment to be incorporated on an ongoing

basis (e.g., the ability to add and/or retire questions, methods, and sources).

4. Estimated costs for conducting each evaluation activity contained within the plan are compared to the actual cost to implement the activity.

5. Strategies such as engineering cost analysis are utilized to examine initial and continuing, as well as alternative, approaches to evaluating.

6. Gantt Charts are used to compare estimated time with actual time required to implement activities.

7. Mechanisms are provided at the time of reporting for those involved to offer suggestions for improvement in the activity the next time it is implemented, as well as to suggest needed changes in questions addressed by the activity.

8. A mechanism for recording decisions resulting from each activity is provided to allow reaction from the audience regarding the utility of the findings for decision making.

In addition, internal evaluators in monitoring the implementation of the plan, as a whole, use this input in aggregate form to examine the effectiveness and efficiency of the evaluation effort across activities and over time. Consider the following:

1. Engineering cost analysis results are considered across activities to provide information regarding those activities that are more or less costly, then compared with the information regarding utilization of results by decisionmakers to obtain information regarding the cost-benefit and/or cost-effectiveness across activities, as well as for each activity over time.

2. Gantt Charts are employed to assess the timeliness of the evaluation effort overall and for each activity over time.

3. Relevance of the evaluation is assessed by examining the nature and extent to which evaluation outcomes are utilized in decision making within the evaluation as a whole, and for each activity over time.

4. Responsibility charts are considered overall and for specific activities, to assess efficiency and continuing support for the whole effort and for segments.

5. The nature of the suggestions made by those reporting results is examined to obtain an indication of how well the plan is working over-

all and to assess the adequacy of the designs used across, as well as within, specific evaluation activities.

In addition to these efforts directed toward evaluating the evaluation by participants, provision should be made for evaluation by organization outsiders. Whenever possible, external evaluators should be involved in procedure and product review for specific activities, as appropriate or necessary. Often this can be accomplished relatively inexpensively by mail and/or telephone, using experts in other areas of the organization (or geographically close) who are not involved in the evaluation or in any manner affected by its results. Internal evaluators with credibility and involvement in the nursing profession or evaluation community at large often have networks established for peer review. It is a reciprocal agreement that involves little or no exchange of money.

Distinctions must be made early by evaluation participants regarding what are considered minor and major changes in evaluation activities, and when each type of change is considered. There is a danger of becoming so responsive to ongoing suggestions for change in evaluation processes and procedures that comparability across time in the results of evaluation activities is jeopardized. Also, changes may be made prematurely, resulting in unnecessary increases in cost or reduced validity of the resulting decisions. Cooley (1984), writing about the utilization of evaluation, makes an important point regarding the need to distinguish between the "evaluation being used and the evaluator being used." He emphasizes that if the evaluation activity is guided by the information requirements and needs of a variety of stakeholders with a broad range of interests, the evaluation effort, if it tends to try to serve everyone's needs, may end up serving no one effectively. He points out that while the selection of evaluation problems is guided by the audience's need for information, it is important for the evaluator to remain disciplined with respect to the "rules of evidence," that is, the methods employed. In other words, the evaluators should, if they are well prepared in evaluation, remain the internal experts in how to proceed methodologically. The soundness of their approach should withstand close inspection by their evaluation colleagues, rather than be subject to change on the basis of audience reaction. As noted earlier, unpopular findings and or threats to vested interests too often take the form of criticism of evaluators and/or evaluation processes and procedures. For this reason, suggestions in this sensitive area need close attention before change is made.

It is important during evaluation planning stages to identify when it is most useful, relevant, and timely to consider changes in the process as a whole and/or to make major changes in specific activities, and to schedule external evaluation of the evaluation at that point in time. Meta-evaluation, using external evaluators, can serve many useful purposes. It can be used to verify evaluation design, progress, and results (e.g., an internal evaluation report, when it is accompanied by an external meta-evaluation report, will increase authoritative credibility). Meta-evaluation can also provide the basis for revision of an evaluation design, its ongoing work, or evaluation reports. When the evaluation is already concluded, meta-evaluation can address the validity and credibility of the results, and it helps maintain involvement in the evaluation as well as raise its credibility and authority. Meta-evaluation efforts can range from an extensive verification to a brief consultation visit, and they can be employed whenever the evaluators or evaluation needs assistance. Typically, meta-evaluations are scheduled during the planning stages of the evaluation and at some point during the implementation. When appropriate, they are also scheduled to assess an evaluation upon its completion.

Meta-evaluations are conducted by an external evaluator or evaluation team. If an individual is conducting the meta-evaluation, that person should be most competent in conducting evaluations as well as in judging evaluations and should have credibility with the external audiences. An evaluation team is often employed when an individual with the necessary credentials can't be found, if there are time pressures. Each member of the team is selected for a particular area of expertise. When resources demand that a decision be made regarding an individual or team, Brinkerhoff et al. (1983) suggest that it is more crucial to have an expert in evaluation than an expert in the content area of interest, because meta-evaluation focuses on judging the worth of the evaluation.

The meta-evaluator should be provided with a set of criteria to be used in the evaluation of the evaluation. Criteria include intended goals and purposes, mandates, audience's expectations, adherence to the design or model for evaluating, or criteria established by expert evaluators. As noted earlier, there are standards and criteria available for this purpose, and they include the following: (1) *Standards for Evaluations of Educational Programs, Projects, and Materials* (1981); (2) Joint Dissemination and Review Panel Criteria (Tallmadse, 1977); (3) *Standards for Audits of Governmental Organizations, Programs, Activities, and Functions* (1981); (4) U.S. Office of Special Education and Rehabilitation Services, Handicapped Personnel Preparation Program: Guidelines for Developing/Rating the Adequacy of Program Evaluation Designs Included with Funded Proposals (1981); and (5) NLN Council of Baccalaureate and Higher Degree Programs Self Study Criteria Number 36 (NLN, 1983).

Methods employed in the meta-evaluation can be quite formal or informal. The more the evaluation is structured and a formal report required, the more external credibility will be given to the resulting report. Brinkerhoff et al. (1983) suggest the following methods for conducting meta-evaluations:

1. Checklists.
2. Formal written critiques.
3. Consultant expert reviews.
4. Field tests.
5. Conferences, hearings, panels.
6. Presentations at professional meetings.
7. Comparisons with other evaluations.
8. Verification studies.
9. Reanalysis.
10. Spot checks of data analysis, information collection procedures, etc.
11. Interviews with respondents.
12. Document reviews.
13. Product reviews.
14. Publication in journals with critiques.

In Waltz's view, an evaluation should be comprehensive but cost-efficient (1985), and, thus, when her approach is employed, it is important that the evaluation of the evaluation focus on cost as it impacts on decision making. The evaluation must not be allowed to become an end in its own right. Furthermore, in her approach to evaluation, the success of the evaluation depends heavily on the quality of the resulting decisions.

Weiner, Rubin, and Sachse (1977) proposed the following three types of impact or influence that evaluations can have: allocative, symbolic, and appreciative. *Allocative influence*, that desired by most evaluators, is when the results of the evaluation affect ". . . discrete, authoritative actions concerning changes in program budgets, formation and enforcement of regulations, modifications of organizational structure, and decisions about expansion, continuation, or cancellation of specific program components" (p. 3). *Symbolic influence* is described by Weiner and colleagues as that

> ... occurring when the existence of an evaluation serves a ritual function, and its success is independent of the message the evaluation brings to decision-makers. The perceived legitimacy of organizations sponsoring evaluation and, hence, their stability, is enhanced when commissioning of an evaluation reassures people that the program under evaluation is being taken seriously. Further, the act of evaluation implies a promise that program changes will be based upon the evaluation results. (p. 2)

Weiner notes this type of evaluation appears to be far more prevalent than evaluators and those commissioning evaluations would like to admit. *Appreciative influence* has a threefold aspect: First, it is akin to power-brokering through distribution of information, which leads to a change of political weights for different forms of evidence. This often tends to enhance the political weight of the evaluator and devalue that of others. The second is influence on people's perceptions of program purposes, i.e., their perceptions of the desirability and/or legitimacy of program goals. The third type is that affecting opinions concerning alternative program strategies—influence that shapes people's ideas about which strategies are most productive. There are situations in which one or more of these influences will be intended by those commissioning the evaluation. In other situations, the same influences may well be unintended outcomes of the evaluation. Some of the influences come from the use of the findings, and others are due to the process.

Whether intended or unintended, these influences represent some of the dimensions of impact to which evaluators must attend in planning, conducting, and evaluating an evaluation. To ignore these consequences would be naive, and the evaluation of the evaluation components incomplete, unless these influences are taken into account. In the Waltz approach, allocative influence is an important indicator of successful evaluation.

SUMMARY

This chapter presents a discussion of the specific steps undertaken when the Waltz approach is employed for the evaluation of nursing programs. Discussion is organized in terms of: (1) who is responsible for the evaluation; (2) why the evaluation is conducted, (3) what is evaluated, (4) how judgments are made on the basis of findings, (5) how the evaluation proceeds, (6) when evaluation occurs, (7) reporting and recording findings and results, and (8) evaluating the evaluation. Specific strategies and techniques for developing and implementing the Master Plan for Evaluation and for managing the conduct of the ongoing evaluation are described. Specific topics regarding "who" include the following: establishing and maintaining the internal evaluator role, operationalizing the internal evaluator role, ethical and political aspects of the role, essential characteristics of internal evaluators, maintaining an outsider perspective in the insider role, and determining significant others to be involved. In the section on "why," attention is given to explaining the purposes for the evaluation and identifying the potential audiences for results. Regarding "what," the focus is on examining program inputs, processes, outcomes, and the setting in which the evaluation occurs, rendering goals and objectives measurable, and explicating questions of concern to the respective audiences. Attention in the section on "how" emphasizes the following: establishing a procedure for decision making, constructing a variable matrix, categorizing evaluation activities, assigning responsibility for evaluation activities using responsibility charting, determining the cost of evaluation activities via engineering cost analysis, and establishing priorities. Gantt Charts are discussed in terms of "when," and essential components and considerations in reporting and recording are elaborated. Meta-evaluation, evaluating the evaluation, is discussed as it relates to the Master Plan, the implementation of specific activities, and strategies and techniques for managing the evaluation.

REFERENCES

Alkin, M. C. (1980). Naturalistic study of evaluation utilization. *New Directions for Program Evaluation, 5,* 19–28.

Brinkerhoff, R. O., Brethower, D. M., Hluchyj, T., & Nowakowski, J. R. (1983). *Program evaluation: Sourcebook casebook.* Boston: Klumer-Nijhoff Publishing.

Campbell, D. T. (1963). Social attitudes and other acquired behavioral dispositions. In S. Koch (Ed.), *Psychology: A study of a science,* Vol. 6. New York: McGraw-Hill.

Comptroller General of the United States. (1981). *Standards for audit of governmental organizations, programs activities and functions.* Washington, DC: U.S. Government Printing Office.

Cooley, W. M. (1984). The difference between the evaluation being used and the evaluator being used. In S. J. Hueftle (Ed.), *The utilization of evaluation proceedings of the 1983 Minnesota evaluation conference* (pp. 27–40). Minnesota: Minnesota Research & Evaluation Center.

Gagne, R. M. (1962). The acquisition of knowledge. *Psychological Review, 69,* 355.

Guttentug, M. (Ed). (1977). *Evaluation studies: Review annual, vol. 2.* Beverly Hills: Sage.

Hart, S., & Waltz, C. (1988). *Educational outcomes: Assessment of quality—state of the art and future directions.* New York: National League for Nursing.

Helmer, O. (1966). *Social technology.* New York: Basic Books.

Joint Committee on Standards for Educational Evaluation. (1981). *Standards for evaluations of educational programs, projects, and materials.* New York: Mc-Graw-Hill.

Lindeman, C. (1975). Delphi survey of providers in clinical nursing research. *Nursing Research, 24*(6), 434–441.

Moscovici, I., Armstrong, P., Shortell, S., & Bennett, R. (1978). Health services research for decision-makers: The use of the delphi technique to determine health priorities. *Journal of Health Politics, Policy and Law, 2,* 388–409.

National League for Nursing Criteria for the Approval of Baccalaureate and Higher Degree Programs in Nursing. (1983). New York: National League for Nursing.

Salasin, S. (1980). The evaluator as an agent of change. *New Directions for Program Evaluation, 7,* 1–9.

Scriven, M. (1975). Evaluation bias and its control. *The Evaluation Center Occasional Paper Series,* Paper No. 4, Western Michigan University.

Sieber, J. E. (1980). Being ethical: Progressional and personal decisions in program evaluation, *New Directions for Program Evaluation, 7,* 51–61.

Sloan, A. P. (1978). *Coping with inter-unit conflict—conflict management and responsibility charting.* Working Paper. School of Management, Massachusetts Institute of Technology, Cambridge, MA.

Staropoli, C., & Waltz, C. F. (1978). *Developing and evaluating educational programs for health care providers.* Philadelphia: F. A. Davis.

Strickland, O. L., & Waltz, C. F. (1981). The role of the internal program evaluator within an educational setting. Paper presented at Evaluation Network/Evaluation Research Society Joint Meeting, Austin, TX.

Stufflebeam, D. L. (1979). Meta evaluation: A topic of professional and public interest. In *Educational evaluation methodology: The state of the art.* Washington, DC: Second Annual Johns Hopkins University National Symposium on Educational Research.

Tallmadse, S. K. (1977). *Joint dissemination review panel ideabook.* Washington, DC: U.S. Government Printing Office.

Thompson, M. S., Rothrock, J. K., Strain, R., & Palmer, R. H. (1981). Cost analysis for program evaluation. In R. F. Conner (Ed.), *Methodological advances in evaluation research* (pp. 31–46). Beverly Hills: Sage.

University of Maryland. (1986). Strategic Plan. University of Maryland School of Nursing.

U.S. Department of Education. (1981). *Application of grants under handicapped personnel preparation program*. Washington, DC: U.S. Department of Education.

Ventura, M., & Walegora-Serafin, B. (1981, June). Setting priorities for nursing research. *The Journal of Nursing Administration*, 30–34.

Waltz, C. F., Strickland, O. L., & Lenz, E. R. (1984). *Measurement in nursing research*. Philadelphia: F. A. Davis Company.

Waltz, C. F., & Hart, S. (1988). *Measurement of nursing education outcomes: State of the art*. New York: National League for Nursing.

Waltz, C., & Bausell, B. (1981). *Nursing research, design, statistics and computer analysis*. Philadelphia: F. A. Davis Company.

Waltz, C., & Bond, S. (1985). How can a program evaluation be comprehensive and yet cost efficient? *Journal of Nursing Education, 6*(24), 258–261.

Weiner, S., Rubin, D., & Sachse, T. (1977). Pathology in institutional structures for evaluation. Unpublished manuscript, Stanford University, Stanford Evaluation Consortium, Stanford, California.